AN ESSAY
ON THE
ANTIQUITY OF HINDOO MEDICINE
INCLUDING AN
INTRODUCTORY LECTURE
TO THE COURSE OF
MATERIA MEDICA AND THERAPEUTICS,
DELIVERED AT KING'S COLLEGE

AN ESSAY

ON THE

ANTIQUITY OF HINDOO MEDICINE

INCLUDING AN

INTRODUCTORY LECTURE

TO THE COURSE OF

MATERIA MEDICA AND THERAPEUTICS,

DELIVERED AT KING'S COLLEGE

BY

J. F. ROYLE, M.D., F.R. & L.S., SEC. G.S.

LATE OF THE MEDICAL STAFF OF THE BENGAL ARMY,
MEMBER OF THE ASIATIC, THE MEDICAL AND PHYSICAL
SOCIETIES OF CLACUTTA, OF THE
ROYAL MEDICAL SOCIETY OF EDINBURGH,
AND OF THE MEDICO-CHISURGICAL SOCIETY OF
LONDON; &C.
PROFESSOR OF MATERIA MEDICA AND THERAPEUTICS,
KING'S COLLEGE, LONDON.

GYAN

Published by

GYAN

Gyan Publishing House
5, Ansari Road
Daryaganj, New Delhi-110002
Phone: 011-47034999, 9811692060
E-mail: books@gyanbooks.com

Distribution Network
gyanbooks.com
India, USA, Canada, UK, Australia, France

ISBN : 978-81-212-2239-6 (HB)
First Published, 1837

2nd Impression 2021

Printed at: Gyan Press, Delhi.

An Essay on the Antiquity of Hindoo Medicine
Author: J. F. Royle

AN ESSAY

ON THE

ANTIQUITY OF HINDOO MEDICINE,

INCLUDING AN

INTRODUCTORY LECTURE

TO THE COURSE OF

MATERIA MEDICA AND THERAPEUTICS,

DELIVERED AT KING'S COLLEGE.

—◆—

BY

J. F. ROYLE, M.D., F.R. & L.S., SEC. G.S.,

LATE OF THE MEDICAL STAFF OF THE BENGAL ARMY,
MEMBER OF THE ASIATIC, THE MEDICAL AND PHYSICAL SOCIETIES OF CALCUTTA, OF THE ROYAL MEDICAL SOCIETY OF EDINBURGH,
AND OF THE MEDICO-CHIRURGICAL SOCIETY OF LONDON; &c.

PROFESSOR OF MATERIA MEDICA AND THERAPEUTICS,
KING'S COLLEGE, LONDON.

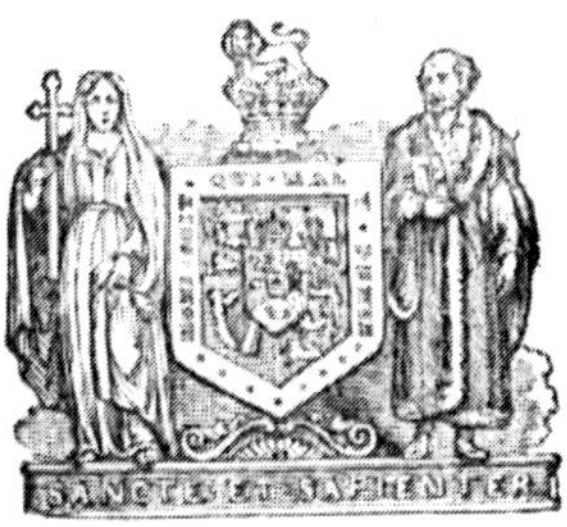

LONDON:

WM. H. ALLEN & Co., 7, Leadenhall Street; and
J. CHURCHILL, Princes Street.

1837.

DEDICATED

TO THE

UNIVERSITY OF MUNICH,

AS A MARK

OF THE

HIGH RESPECT AND GRATEFUL FEELING

OF

THE AUTHOR.

ADVERTISEMENT.

As some incongruity is obvious between the title and the commencement of the present publication, it is advisable to state how it has originated. The Author, on entering on the course of Materia Medica and Therapeutics in King's College, having been requested by his colleagues, as well as some distinguished members of the Profession, to print his Introductory Address, and by others to give proofs of his opinions more in detail; determined, in complying with the former, to attend as much as possible to the latter request. From the pressure of other occupations, it was not until the greater part of the Lecture was in print that the additions (with a few exceptions, those from p. 40 to 192) were made, and at a time, when a publication to the extent it has now reached was never contemplated. The object, in some of these additions, having been to show the probability of the antiquity of Hindoo Medicine in connection with Indian commerce, independent of the proofs afterwards adduced, some repetition will perhaps appear to have been unnecessarily introduced; this was in some measure inseparable from the cumulative nature of the argument adopted, in proceeding from comparatively modern to more ancient times; but partly caused by the interruptions, amidst which this essay has been written. These circumstances are mentioned in hopes of obtaining the reader's consideration, as well as to account for the imperfections of the work, in connection with its title. This has been adopted in conformity to the suggestion of valued friends, that the object of the publication should occupy a more prominent position than its occasion.

62, Berners Street,
1st *January* 1838.

By the same Author:

ILLUSTRATIONS of the BOTANY and other BRANCHES of the NATURAL HISTORY of the HIMALAYAN MOUNTAINS, and of the FLORA of CASHMERE.

Parts I. to IX., imp. 4to., 20s. each, with Coloured Plates.—Part X. will be published shortly.

CONTENTS.

In commencing a course of lectures, it is usual to give some account of the origin and history, the objects and uses of the subject to be entered upon, by teacher and student. The practice has its advantages, in many respects, for all ought to be acquainted both with the object and the use of any study they are about to commence; but few can be interested about the history of a subject with which they are supposed to be totally unacquainted. Though a lecturer may usually choose any part of his subject for his introductory discourse, there are occasions when he feels it expedient to give his own views on the subject to be studied. As I consider that to be my case, I shall enter at once into a consideration of the objects of Materia Medica and Therapeutics, and the sciences with which they are connected, and without which they cannot be understood; adding a short survey of the history of the science, and concluding with some observations on the modes and means of teaching.

Materia Medica treats of the nature in general of medicines, and Therapeutics of their application in the treatment of disease. 'All substances which are applied to diseased organs, with a view to cure or relieve, and which possess this virtue, independent of their nutritive qualities, are medicines.' They are obtained from both the Organic and Inorganic kingdoms, *i.e.* from the Vegetable and Animal, as well as from the Mineral kingdom. It is necessary, therefore, to be acquainted with the sciences which treat of these as objects of Natural history.

Vegetables and their products appear so naturally connected with the healing art, that one of the gods of the East is represented (having assumed the character of a chief physician), as delivering his instructions on the doctrines of medicine, in a forest of medical plants, in the presence of gods, sages, and a large train of both orthodox and heretical hearers. Certainly as plants yielded some of the earliest, so they continue to afford many of the most valuable articles of the Materia Medica of every country of the globe; and the science of vegetation therefore is one of those most closely connected with our subject. Whether we consider the vast variety of beautiful objects brought under review; or the interesting nature of the information which we obtain, by examining into the structure, functions, and properties of each; or the value of the inferences which may be deduced, as applicable to medicine, agriculture, or the arts; there are few that can be compared with it either in variety or value. This statement may appear overstrained to many who have been in the habit of regarding Botany as a science of names only; but it can be so accounted by those alone who, not considering that a multitude of natural objects must necessarily be distinguished by an equal number of names, are appalled by the apparently insurmountable difficulties, and never look from names to the things they indicate. As if a stranger, on entering the vestibule of one of our modern museums, should, from a view of the dilapidated monuments and illegible inscriptions of antiquity, pronounce at once upon their uselessness, because he himself was unable in the one to decipher the history of past times, or to read in the other the mind and design of the sculptor or architect.

But we have not to examine the objects of Botany, nor to

study the structure and functions of plants; nor have we to note the first appearances of life in conjunction with the simplest states of organised cellular matter, to its further development in Endogenous life; where vascular bundles, though performing the same functions, are only bound together, but have not attained that higher degree of centralisation in which the different systems unite into different organs; as the cellular into pith, bark, and medullary rays, and the vascular into rings of wood. Neither have we to watch the local circulation in the cells, nor to trace the more general progression of the sap from the roots to the leaves, and from these downwards into the bark. But we are interested in the laws of vegetable physiology, that we may be able to weigh the influence of the various stimulants of light, heat, air, and moisture; the effects of soils and aspects; that we may understand something of their operation, in modifying the products of plants, and be able to select our barks, woods, and roots, bulbs, leaves, flowers, and fruits, at the age and season when they contain the principles which render them useful as medicines in their most abundant and efficient state; whether these be gums, fecula, or saccharine principle; milky juice or resin; fixed or volatile oil; or any of those numerous alcaloids which are so completely altering the forms of medicines, since the subtleties of modern chemistry discovered them to be secreted in nature's nicer laboratory.

There are, however, two branches of this extensive science, respecting which I am desirous of making a few observations; one is the connexion between the Structure and Natural affinities of plants, and their Physical and Medical properties; and the other is their Geographical distribution, especially as connected with Climate. Both are important subjects, whether we consider them in a scientific or a practical point of view. The one teaches us the laws which influence the distribution of plants;

points out the countries and climates which different families affect; and gives us principles for their cultivation, either as medicines, or as objects of agriculture: the other is no less valuable in affording us innumerable indications in every part of the world, for discovering the properties of new and unknown plants, whether as fitting them for food, for medicine, or for any of the arts of life; and though there are no doubt exceptions, (fewer, however, than usually adduced) there certainly is no other method by which we may so readily find a substitute for a medicine, or an equivalent for an article of trade, as by seeking for it in the families of plants, which are already known to contain some possessed of such properties as we desiderate. This is no trivial advantage; for though our Pharmacopœias and Dispensatories may be models of what is requisite for civilized society, yet if it be considered that the English Schools of Medicine supply practitioners for an empire, on which, without hyperbole, it has been said, the sun never sets; it will readily be allowed, that we may frequently be placed where there are neither chemists to analyse, nor herbalists to select the plants, secreting most valuable products at our feet; but to which we might readily be led by studying their natural affinities. Our systems of Materia Medica might therefore inculcate these more comprehensive doctrines, and a teacher extend the range of his influence and usefulness, while describing any officinal species, by introducing it with general observations on the family to which it belongs, as well as the countries where this is chiefly found. An Indian sage, after giving a prescription of precious stones, for curing the diseases of kings and rich men, very judiciously adds another, for people in general, composed of vegetables, because these are procurable by all.

The system of arrangement, however, alone applicable

to this purpose, is that called the Natural method, which, enabling us to discuss questions concerning the structure of its several groups, in conjunction with climate, geographical distribution, medical and physical properties, makes modern botany a highly interesting and philosophical study. The artificial system of Linnæus, usually taught in this country, is ill adapted for our purpose, and for the present state of science. But I am very far from wishing, by such an observation, to reflect in any manner upon the character or merits of Linnæus, one of the greatest naturalists that ever lived; than whom no one has more strongly expressed the necessity of establishing a more philosophical arrangement, which he considered the ultimate object of study; and who did Natural History the highest services by the invention of methods of arrangement, which prevented its being overwhelmed by the very magnitude of the exertions made in its service. But it is necessary to place the natural classification in a proper point of view, since even one of our principal botanists seemed to think the natural subordinate to the artificial method of classification. In criticising a work of Mr. Robert Brown, who is acknowledged by all Europe as the first Botanist of his day, Sir James Smith says, "He himself will surely not reckon it complete, without a Linnæan Index, 'to give the precious metal sterling worth:' we have done this, Gentlemen, without the Index, by returning, if I may be allowed the expression, from a paper to a golden currency."

The connexion between the medical properties of plants and their structure, was a subject which attracted the attention of botanists at an early period. Thus Cæsalpinus, in 1583, in the Preface to his work, "De Plantis," says, "Quæ enim generis societate junguntur, plerumque et similes possident facultates;" while Camerarius, in 1699, wrote a dissertation, entitled "De Convenientiâ Plantarum in fructificatione et viribus;" Petiver, an apothecary of Aldersgate-street, and well known as a botanist, has a paper in the 21st volume of the Philosophical Transactions (1699), entitled, "Some attempts to prove that herbs of the same make and class, for the generality, have the like virtue, and tendency to work the same effects." Again, Linnæus has stated, "Plantæ quæ Genere conveniunt, etiam virtute conveniunt; quæ Ordine naturali continentur, etiam virtute proprius accedunt; quæque Classi naturali congruunt, etiam viribus quodammodo congruunt." But the progress was inconsiderable in the path pointed out by these illustrious naturalists, until the publication by the celebrated De Candolle, who has thrown a light over so many departments of Botany, of his "Essai sur les propriétés médicales des Plantes." In this work he has shown, that as the effects of the different substances used as medicines, must be owing either to their physical characters or their chemical composition, so must these depend on the peculiar organization of the vegetable, especially in the organs of nutrition, by which they are secreted. But as plants are classified from their organs of reproduction, and not from those of nutrition, it does not appear how we are led to the nature of the secretions formed by these, from a consideration of groupings founded on the examination of a different set of organs. To this it has been well replied, that though an artificial arrangement may draw its characters of classes from as small a number of organs as possible, the natural method is, on the contrary, the more perfect in proportion that the characters of its classes express a greater number of ideas; hence those families which present the most numerous points of analogy in the organs of reproduction, will also display them in the organs of nutrition, in which the secretions are chiefly performed. Thus the division of vegetables from the seeds, into Acotyledons,

Monocotyledons, and Dicotyledons, agrees with that taken from the absence, the existence, and disposition of a vascular system. Hence the peculiarities of the organs of reproduction may be a sufficiently certain index of the structure of those of nutrition; but as these determine the nature of the secretions or products of plants, so it follows that the properties of plants may be in accordance with their classification into natural families.

But as examples are more convincing than general reasoning, we may readily refer to numerous instances, to render this conclusive. No one is surprised at hearing that the *Gramineæ* of tropical regions are as fitted for food as those of European countries; or that the oak of the Himalaya yields excellent timber; or that pines abound in turpentine, and may be made to yield tar wherever they are found. So the *Rosaceæ* afford us our best fruits; among the *Papilionaceæ*, are found all the legumes used as food in different parts of the world, and the *Labiatæ* yield most of our odoriferous herbs, as lavender, rosemary, thyme, sage, savory, marjoram, and mint. The *Burseraceæ*, a tribe of *Terebinthaceæ*, afford resins combined with essential oil; as we see in the balm of Gilead and Myrrh trees, *Balsamodendron gileadense* and *Myrrha; B. opobalsamum*, *Kataf* and *Kalaf*, all give out a balsamic odour. Indian Bdellium is probably produced by *Balsamodendron Agallocha;* African Bdellium is yielded by another of this family, *Heudelotia africana;* Olibanum by *Boswellia serrata; Pistacia Terebinthus* and *Lentiscus*, afford us Chio turpentine and Mastic. The *Laurels* give us the Camphor of Japan; the Cinnamon of China, as well as that of Ceylon; Cassia, Sindoc, Calitlawan, the Malabathrum leaf in India, and the Bay-leaf in Europe. Of the *Dipterocarpeæ*, one species yields the Camphor of Sumatra; *Shorea robusta* the resin called *ral*, but *dammer* by the English; while *Vateria indica* produces copal, and *Dipterocarpus costatus, turbinatus, incanus, alatus*, and probably other species, afford the balsam called Wood-oil. So many of the *Guttiferæ* exude a gamboge-like substance, that we may safely conclude the officinal species, though unknown, to be of this family; as also that the Officinal Rhubarb, though equally unknown, is yielded by a species of *Rheum;* and as the *Umbelliferæ* give us Assafœtida, Galbanum, Opoponax, and Ammoniacum, we infer that they also afford us Sagapenum.

The *Cedrelaceæ* are remarkable for their bitterness and astringency, accompanied frequently by an aromatic principle; and thence are endowed with febrifuge properties. So *Soymida febrifuga,* with others, is reckoned in India a good stomachic and febrifuge; the *Khaya* is similarly employed on the banks of the Gambia; *Cedrela febrifuga* in Java, and *Swietenia Mahogani* in the New World. As we thence get Logwood and Brazil wood, so from the Malayan Peninsula we have Sappan wood, all from the *Cæsalpineæ.* Of the *Memispermaceæ, Cocculus palmatus* affords the well-known Columba root; but in India, *C. cordifolius* is no less extensively employed as a tonic and febrifuge; so the Brazilians employ *Cocculus platyphyllus, cinerascens,* and *ovalifolius,* for the cure of intermittent fevers; as do the Malays in Eastern countries, *C. peltatus, crispus,* and *Fibraurea.* The *Gentianeæ* not only yield bitter roots and herbs in Europe, as gentian and centaury, but in the Himalayas they afford us *Gentiana Kurroa* as a bitter root, and the *Cheretta* as a herb.

The *Nima* of these mountains is as bitter as the Quassia of South America, and both belong to the family of *Simarubeæ.* The *Solaneæ* are well known for their narcotic properties, as exhibited in several solanums, the henbane, datura, and deadly night-shade. Among the *Cinchonaceæ*, the true Cinchonas are too well known for their febrifuge properties to require further notice, except that in proportion to the number of species yielding medicinal bark, is the difficulty of assigning to any particular species, those kinds which are officinal. But in countries where the true Cinchonas do not exist, others of this family are used as substitutes, as *Pinckneya pubens* in Carolina, *Portlandia hexandra* in French Guiana, *Rondeletia febrifuga* in Sierra Leone; so also *Macrocnemum corymbosum*, *Guettarda coccinea*, *Antirrhœa verticillata*, *Morinda Royoc*, and others; with *Hymenodictyon excelsum* in India.

Of the *Convolvulaceæ*, *Ipomœa Jalapa* of Nuttal yields the true jalap, and *Convolvulus Scammonia*, scammony; so in India, *Ipomœa Turpethum* forms the *toorbud* of the Arabs, probably corrupted from the Sanscrit *trivrit*; and the seeds of *Ipomœa cœrulea*, described by Mesue under the name of *hub-al-nil* and *granum indicum*, are still used in India for their purgative properties. In the *Cucurbitaceæ* there exists a bitter principle in the fruit of many species; and in the rind of the cucumber and the melon. Of this family, colocynth, squirting cucumber, and bryony, are used as purgatives; in India, with the true colocynth, there is a nearly allied species substituted for it, which I have named *Cucumis pseudo-Colocynthis*; some other species of this genus, as well as of *Trichosanthes*, *Luffa*, and *Lagenaria*, are likewise used as purgatives.

In connexion with this subject may be mentioned a discovery to which I was led, entirely by inferences drawn from the natural affinities of plants. In a paper lately read to the British Association at Bristol, on the plants which yielded Caoutchouc, I observed that they all belonged to the milky-juiced families of *Cichoraceæ*, *Lobeliaceæ*, *Apocyneæ*, *Asclepiadeæ*, *Euphorbiaceæ*, and *Artocarpeæ*, a tribe of *Urticeæ*. In the first place, it may be observed that many of the plants of these families are remarkable for the strength and tenacity of the fibre they yield for rope-making: secondly, that bird-lime is prepared from plants belonging to families which yield caoutchouc, as from the apocyneous Voacanga in Madagascar; and in India, from different species of *Ficus* and *Artocarpus*. But the most interesting fact which I obtained from the investigation, was one most unexpected, and the least connected with the subject. Having been previously employed in considering the proper means for extending the cultivation of silk in India; it struck me as singular, that so many of the plants which silk-worms prefer next to the mulberry leaf, should be found in those families which yield caoutchouc. Thus, in England, the lettuce and dandelion leaves, belonging to *Cichoraceæ*, and in India *Ficus religiosa*, belonging to the *Artocarpeæ*, have been ascertained to be the best substitutes for the leaves of the mulberry; while the Arindy silk-worm of India, *Phalæna Cynthia*, feeds upon those of the castor oil plant, *Ricinus communis*, belonging to *Euphorbiaceæ*.* Considering that a circumstance of this nature was not likely to be accidental, I was induced to think that it depended upon the presence of some principle common to all these vegetables, and therefore that caoutchouc (perhaps in a modified state) might really be contained in the juice of the mulberry, though this is described as not being milky. I therefore requested Mr. Sievier, who has made so many discoveries in the properties of caoutchouc, to ascertain whether my conjecture was well founded. In a

* Since this lecture was delivered, I have seen in the newspapers, that a species of *Scorzonera*, which belongs to the natural family of *Cichoraceæ*, has been found to be a good substitute for the mulberry-leaf in France. I have also been informed by Mr. Morley, that a caterpillar which forms a very large cacoon, and spins a tough but coarse kind of silk, feeds on the leaves of the South American caoutchouc-tree, *Siphonia elastica*.

few days he informed me that the mulberry-tree sap was of a milky nature, and did actually contain caoutchouc, especially on dry and bright sunny days.

With respect to the Geographical distribution of Plants, especially in its connexion with Climate, I wish to say a few words, in order to shew that the argument I afterwards draw from it, is based on a sure foundation. In repeating nearly what I have said elsewhere,. I shall confine myself to the more marked differences of climate, and the vegetation it supports.

The peculiarities of the tropical zone we well know to be brightness of light, great heat, and moisture, with considerable uniformity of all throughout the year. These are all favourable to the development of vegetation, whicn is accordingly characterised by vastness; the foliage, by richness; and the inflorescence, by brilliancy of colouring. Hence, the proportion of trees is great, and their flowers of a size and richness which, in colder climates, are only the appanage of humbler plants; as may be seen in the noble Amherstia, the wide-spreading Bombax, or glowing Erythrina. If we study the physiology of plants, as well as the circumstances controlling their growth, and the nature of their secretions, we find that vegetation is much affected by the different physical states of the soil and atmosphere, as well as by the supply of heat and light; hence we may conclude, that there are different sets of plants fitted by nature for the particular circumstances in which they are to be placed. Those who have visited tropical countries, know that the position of their low and mangrove-lined coasts may be recognised by the forests of tall palms, shooting like distant masts above the surface of the sea. The very mention of the Clove, the Cinnamon, Nutmeg, Ginger, Cardamom, Plantain and Pepper recall ideas of high temperature and rich vegetation: but these all belong to separate families of plants, as *Myrtaceæ*,

Lauraceæ, *Myristiceæ*, *Scitamineæ*, *Musaceæ*, and *Piperaceæ*, which prevail in equatorial forests, and perfectly characterise tropical vegetation; but they do not do so more than the *Anonaceæ*, *Dilleniaceæ*, *Guttiferæ*, *Aurantiaceæ*, *Dipterocarpeæ*, *Sapindaceæ*, *Meliaceæ*, *Combretaceæ*, *Cinchonaceæ*, *Bignoniaceæ*, *Ebenaceæ*, *Sapoteæ*, *Cycadaceæ*, *Bromeliaceæ*, *Pandanaceæ*, and many others. As tropical climate is not terminated by an abrupt line, but, according to the influence of local causes, extended into higher latitudes, so does it carry with it the peculiarities of tropical vegetation. Thus, if the country be open towards the equator, the equinoctial rains will be blown with the periodical winds to much higher latitudes than where a mountain range intervenes, or the course of the winds is diverted by a high and shelving coast. Hence India, open to the south, is deluged by the periodical rains; while Egypt, in the same latitude, owes its fertility only to the overflowing of the Nile. The same effects may ensue, if the same causes operate, along a valley or a mountain range. Thus, Humboldt has shewn that, in the basin of the Ohio, *Gleditsia monosperma*, the *Catalpa*, and *Aristolochia Sipho*, extend three degrees further north than on the coast of the Atlantic. So, along the base of the Himalayas, where there is considerable moisture of the soil, a vigorous vegetation has sprung up, which adds to the humidity of the atmosphere, as well by exhalation from its leaves as by preventing free evaporation from the ground. A greater equality of temperature is also preserved, from the umbrageous covering at once impeding the ready absorption of heat by day, as it checks free radiation during the night. Hence, along this tropic-girt base, with greater equability of temperature, we find more uniform moisture than in the open plains; and in it many plants extending several degrees further north than they do in any other part of India; as, a species of *Cinna-*

momum, yielding the *tej-pat*, or bay-leaf of India, the *Malabathrum* of the Ancients; also *Piper longum*, which does not, however, furnish long pepper sufficiently good or abundantly enough to be an article of commerce; together with *Shorea robusta*, one of the *Dipterocarpeæ; Embryopteris glutinifera*, one of the *Ebenaceæ;* as well as *Semecarpus Anacardium*, and the Catechu-yielding *Acacia;* with *Bauhinia racemosa* and *Hiptage Madablota*, as gigantic climbers. Here the geologist will be interested in seeing a full-grown Pine alongside of a dwarfish Palm, and the Rattan trailing in valleys, with the Plantain wild and flourishing at the foot of mountains, on which species of *Acer, Ulmus, Betula, Carpinus*, and *Juglans* (genera found in a fossil state) are growing in fullest luxuriance. The agriculturalist will here notice the excellence of the rice cultivated in some of these vallies, and that the Banana, Jack-fruit (*Artocarpus integrifolia*), and Guava (*Psidium pyriferum*) succeed nearly as well as in the rich soil and moist climate of Bengal.

If we wish, however, to draw either scientific or practical deductions from the prevalence in any situation of particular plants, we must pay especial attention on the one hand to the habit, and on the other to the proportional number of the species, as compared with the general character of the family; for though the different families of plants occur in the greatest numbers in particular countries and climates, yet they frequently send their representatives into very distant regions. Thus we have in the south of Europe, either indigenous or introduced, a Laurel, a Palm, a Myrtle, Oleander, Calotropis, Vitex, and a few Acacias, all which belong to families occurring in the greatest numbers in tropical countries. So, some of those which form the largest trees of Equinoctial regions occur in European countries as annual herbs; as of the *Malvaceæ*, the huge Silk-cotton-tree in the former, and the humble Mallow in the latter; of *Verbenaceæ*, the Teak in India, and the Vervein in Europe; of *Rubiaceæ*, the Cinchona in South America, and the weak Rubia in Europe; and of the *Euphorbiaceæ*, the lowly spurges in European countries, the shrubby *Euphorbias* in the hot parts of Africa and India, and the arboreous species of *Emblica*, *Rottlera*, *Elæococca*, *Stillingia*, and *Siphonia*, in tropical parts of the world.

As the diminution of temperature in the atmosphere is very gradual, according to the elevation; so is the disappearance of tropical forms as we ascend mountains: hence we find such plants diminishing in number and size as we climb either the Andes or the Himalayas. Their existence at considerable heights may probably be favoured by the range of the thermometer being less on mountain tops than on plains, even where the mean temperature is the same; and, perhaps, the effect of the extremes of temperature may be less injurious when transmitted through a more rarefied medium. But in mountains under the influence of tropical rains, a peculiarity of atmosphere occurs analogous to that so well characterised by Baron Humboldt in the Andes, as "the region of clouds." So in the Himalayas, at seven and eight thousand feet of elevation, the thermometer does not vary ten degrees during three months: and even when rain does not fall, there is constant humidity, from the air charged with moisture in the heated valleys rising and depositing it on the mountains, when it reaches an elevation where it is cooled below the point of saturation. The cloudiness, at the same time, preventing the full influence of the sun's rays; and at night the radiation from a mountain ridge bearing but a small proportion to the mass of the atmosphere, comparative little cooling takes place; and the thermometer is but a few degrees lower in the morning than it was on the previous evening: so that the same equability which we have observed at the base of the mountains, takes place at considerable elevations, from the operation of other causes. This being combined with moisture, we have two of the characteristics of a tropical climate, and find that, in such circumstances, a less degree of heat is essential for the maintenance of plants otherwise indicative, though only annuals, of tropical vegetation. Of these may be instanced one of the *Scitamineæ*, the family to which the ginger and cardamom belong, at as great an elevation as nine thousand feet, with Balsams, Begonias, *Cyrtandraceæ*, *Melastomaceæ*, a *Smithia*, *Cassia*, &c.: even a Bamboo is found as high as ten thousand feet; but its annual stems are yearly levelled by the falls of snow, while the roots are protected by their subterranean situation from the great changes of temperature. It is this moist state of the atmosphere, and the frequent showers previous to its accession, which render practicable, at considerable elevations in these mountains, the cultivation of rice; an annual that ripens in a few months. This shews how futile was the attempt to cultivate it in this country, merely because there appeared to those who thought only of temperature, a similarity in climate.

But luxuriant vegetation is not confined to tropical countries, as we know from the beauty and variety of scenery in temperate climes, dependant on an entirely different set of plants. Among these, the *Coniferæ* are conspicuous; and the *Amentaceæ* give the greatest variety of trees, as oaks, chestnuts, birches, horn-beams, hazels, poplars, and willows; with elms, maples, rhododendrons, and the walnut, which, though found in southern latitudes, grow in mountainous situations only. But these are not more indicative of moderate temperature than are many other families of plants; as the *Ranunculaceæ*, *Gentianeæ*, *Primulaceæ*, *Saxifrageæ*, *Valerianeæ*, *Campanulaceæ*, *Rosaceæ*, some tribes of *Labiatæ*, *Cruciferæ*, *Caryo-*

phylleæ, and *Umbelliferæ*. As elevation produces the same effects on temperature as increase of latitude, we find in the Himalayas a climate so suited to these families, that they form the most numerous portion of its flora. In company with them, also, occur some of the plants of China and Japan, as well as of North America; and on the northern face, several of those of Siberia. Many of the lofty peaks being covered with snow for nine months in the year, which melts only when the sun has the greatest power, we may suppose the brightness of light in this thin and rarefied medium, to be an equivalent for the uninterrupted sunshine of polar regions during the same months; and the climate as suited to the growth of plants, which can scarcely be distinguished from some brought from Melville Island. A dwarf willow and birch, with a rhododendron, forming the ligneous vegetation of high latitudes, so does a species of the first, with rhododendrons, occur at the highest elevations in the Himalayas, though the birch exists only as a tree within the limit of forest. In the same way that we have seen tropical families sending a few species into temperate climates, so do those which are characteristic of the latter, send their representatives into the midst of tropical vegetation; but these, with the exception of the multiform willow, are only annuals which spring up, flower, and seed, during the cold-weather months in India; as one or two Gentians; *Anagallis*, of the family of *Primulaceæ; Silene conoidea*, and *Saponaria Vaccaria*, in corn-fields; with *Ranunculus sceleratus* and *aquatilis*, growing in, and near water; therefore able, from its equalising effects, to bear great vicissitudes of atmospheric temperature.

But as these occur only in the cold-weather months, or from October to April, so does the cultivation in these months in the plains of India correspond with that of the summer months of higher latitudes; consisting of wheat, barley, flax, peas, beans, &c. with the culture of the poppy, and the collection of opium, in the very same fields, perhaps, where, in the rainy season, had been grown rice, sorghum, and other tropical grains.

Such are a few general views respecting the Geography of plants in connexion with climate. Between the extreme points of a tropical and a polar vegetation, we might shew a series of gradations: but these would lead into unnecessary detail; and the object has, perhaps, been sufficiently gained, if I have been successful in shewing in what way the distribution of plants is connected with climate; and consequently what is the value of any inferences that may be deduced from their culture in new situations; and also from vegetable products being found in countries where the plants themselves are unable to grow.

The Animal creation is the next which should attract our attention, or at least be considered in connexion with the vegetable kingdom, whether we adopt the ascending or the descending series. Here we find sensibility superadded to the vital principle, which we first saw in union with matter in the lowest forms of organized vegetation. Interesting and instructive as is the study of the forms and habits of the animal world; indispensable as is an acquaintance with their internal structure and functions to a scientific knowledge of the anatomy and physiology of the human frame; these are of comparatively less consequence in a course of Materia Medica: because in proportion as the progress of medicine has brought the art of prescription nearer to its original simplicity, so the crowd of inert and disgusting remedies, introduced by the corrupters of medicine, have disappeared from our pharmacopœias. As animals require for their nutriment matter which has already been organized, either by vegetables or lower grades of animal life, so do they carry it to a higher state of organization, and bring it nearer to the nature of man himself. Hence they are less and less fitted for effecting those changes in the functions and states of organs, which form the objects of medicines; but they are therefore the better suited for affording materials of renovation to the exhausted frame; as we may see by the large proportion of the Vertebrata employed for food. That a greater number of medicines were formerly obtained from the animal kingdom, is not therefore to be ascribed to their powers having been supplanted by a more abundant and perfect supply from the vegetable and mineral kingdoms. But then, the general ignorance of both practitioner and patient allowed the former, by means of loathsome remedies, to operate on the imagination of the latter; in hopes of producing those changes in the state of disease, which his knowledge did not tell him how otherwise to effect. The reign of ignorance is not yet passed; but more elegant modes have been successively devised, for producing the same results; by those who have less excuse than their predecessors for such practices.

The exceptions to the above observation, are but few: musk and castor still continue to be used; but these seem to be secreted by the respective animals for acting as stimulants to some of their own functions: certain substances are employed as emollients, and operate chiefly by their mechanical properties; to these may be added carbonate of lime, secreted in large quantities by lower tribes of animals, as a defence against their numerous enemies; but which the improved state of chemistry has shown, can be procured of equal purity and with greater facility from the mineral kingdom. So few articles being now obtained as medicines from the animal kingdom, it is of less consequence to ascertain whether there be that connexion between structure and its properties, as we have seen to exist in the vegetable kingdom. But if we look at the different kinds of animals employed as food, and those which are not so, we shall see a recognition of the principle; as well as in the employment of several species of the tribe of *Cantharidia*, as vesicatories in different countries.

From viewing the Organic we proceed to the Inorganic kingdom of nature, and Mineralogy, as one great division of natural history, embraces within its consideration the structure and relations of minerals, or all bodies found in or upon the earth, which are neither animal nor vegetable. Crystallography is a branch of this science, which describes and explains the relations that subsist among the crystalline forms of minerals, while Geology makes us acquainted with the structure, relative position, materials, and mode of formation of the mineral masses, of which the crust of the earth is composed. Minerals, though inorganized, act on organized matter, so as to produce those changes in its state and functions, which make them useful as medicines. They may, whether solid, liquid, or aëriform, be arranged and distinguished, either according to their physical characters, or their chemical composition. But few are now employed, either as external or internal remedies, until they have been subjected to some chemical operation, either to improve their quality, or to change their nature. As all that are employed as medicines are also objects of chemistry, it is in every way preferable to treat of them according to the most approved arrangements of this science; introducing, however, in appropriate places, the natural history and physical characters of such as are chiefly the produce of nature. It is indispensable, therefore, that we be acquainted with the sciences which treat of them in this view, to know that we use their terms with propriety and correctness.

But these studies, extensive though they be, and indispensable as it is for us to understand the arrangements which they adopt, and the places which the objects we wish to examine occupy in the scheme of nature, do not embrace all that is requisite respecting the substances we have to employ as medicines, even independent of their uses as such. For those which we find most useful as remedies may occupy little of the attention of the naturalist; as we only employ them when they have ceased to be of use to the objects of his care; or at least they may never engage his notice in the way in which we view them. A knowledge of natural bodies implies also an acquaintance with their physical states and chemical composition. The former consists in the examination of such properties as their hardness, elasticity, specific gravity, powers of electricity or refraction; all principal objects of attention in Natural Philosophy, a science which should form a part, not only of professional, but of general education. As students of medicine, I know not how the admirable mechanism of the human body, the circulation of its fluids, or the effects of atmospherical vicissitudes with respect to temperature, density, or moisture, as affecting especially the functions of respiration and perspiration; or the general effects of light, heat, and electricity on the human system, can be well understood, unless we study these general powers, and see how they control or affect almost every function. For if we do not understand their operation on the animal economy, when in a state of health, we are not likely to do so when we wish to employ them as general remedies in disease. These great powers, heat, light, electricity, and magnetism, come under the cognizance of the chemical, as well as of the natural philosopher, though in somewhat different points of view; the former considering them more as agents effecting changes, and the latter as great principles of nature and powers in motion.

The object of the Chemist being to ascertain the constituents of all bodies, whether animal, vegetable, or mineral; to investigate the way in which these constituents combine, and the nature of the compounds which they form; his science must be admitted as indispensable as any for acquiring an accurate knowledge of natural bodies, more especially if we study them with a view to their employment as medicinal agents. These, as we have said, are seldom administered as afforded by nature, but undergo several operations, some mechanical, others entirely chemical, constituting that branch of study called Pharmacy. For this, we require to be intimately acquainted with the laws of Chemistry, and the mutual action of bodies on each other, that we may not compound what are incongruous, or prescribe such as are incompatible. But the value of this science towards acquiring an accurate knowledge of Materia Medica is too well known to require being insisted on, whether we regard retrospective services or prospective aids. For I feel well assured, looking at the all-pervading grasp of Chemistry, and its recent achievements, that we shall every year be furnished with new agents and new forms, as well from the mineral, as from the vegetable kingdom; more especially if the chemical philosopher will subject to his examination, not only those plants of which the uses are known, but the many others also which invite his attention; and to which he will be best, nay, easily guided, by attending to the Natural affinities of plants.

But the most finished natural-historical description, the most accurate ascertainment of physical properties, the nicest analysis, or the most elegant preparation, form but a small, or, at least, only the preliminary portion of the duties which devolve upon the teacher or student of Materia Medica. For we have still to inquire, what are the Physiological action of medicines, or the changes effected by the substances so called, when applied to the different surfaces of the human body, in health or in disease; whether these changes be of a chemical nature, or owing to some peculiar influence exercised on the vital energy; whether they be local or general, primary or secondary; and whether the substances be carried into the system by absorption, or act by sympathy; attending, at the same time, to all the different circumstances which may modify their action, when administered in disease.

Even this is only the last step of the ladder up which we have been climbing, to reach the ultimate end and object of the whole, which is Therapeutics, or the administration of remedies, for the purpose of removing the tendency to disease, and of inducing a return to a healthy action of the various organs and functions of the body. Every thing, therefore, capable of effecting such objects, is called to his aid by the Therapeutist, whether they be of the class usually called Medicines, or come under the more comprehensive denomination of Remedies, whether these be Physical or Moral agents. Materia Medica, therefore, instead of being on an equality with Therapeutics, must ever be considered as secondary and subordinate, "non soror, sed ancilla," a handmaiden only, not a sister, bringing together, preparing, and trying whatever may be likely to fulfil the indications, which the other, informed by the higher course of pathological study, has ascertained to be necessary for the removal of disease. Medicine is therefore connected with other sciences through Therapeutics, which we have seen cannot be successfully practised, without, on the one hand, a knowledge of Pathology, or the doctrines of disease, and on the other, an acquaintance with Materia Medica, or the nature and actions of medicines. As M.M. Trousseau and Pidoux, the most recent authors, and of high authority, are of opinion, that all writers give too much attention to Materia Medica, and too little to Therapeutics, we must endeavour, in our observations on each article, as well as on each class of remedies, to avoid, if possible, incurring this reproach; without, however, encroaching on the province of the Professor of Medicine.

Such are the several Sciences connected with the various articles of Materia Medica. These, it will be needless, nay, impossible, to enumerate. Such as are now in use, will, of course, be the objects of our special attention. Those which have ceased to be so, or have not yet become generally established, may, without entering into details, serve to establish a principle, or elucidate the works of some of the masters in medicine. Under each of the former, we shall have to attend both to its Natural History characters, its Physical properties, Chemical composition, Physiological effects, and Therapeutical uses, as well as its Pharmaceutical preparations, and its Literary and Commercial history. The last, in a country like Great Britain, it would be supposed must be both correct and easy to procure; but it will generally be found that traders care little, except about the price of a drug, and the port where it may be purchased; and brokers, in this country, think only of the ship in which it was imported, and the place whence this was cleared; though the substance itself may have been first conveyed thither from very distant regions. We shall be led, therefore, to a geographical inquiry into the countries where our drugs are produced. America, the latest discovered, may be most quickly dismissed, as comparatively less complicated in the commercial history of its products; though from the unequalled extent of territory, and great diversity of climate, it supplies almost every variety of medicinal agent, and among them many of our most valuable drugs, as bark, ipecacuanha, jalap, &c. The

Old World, however, is equally varied in its treasures, whether we look to such as require a cold or temperate climate with moisture, as almost every part of Europe; or such as are only elaborated in the bright skies and sunny climes of the Mediterranean or Persian regions. Others again refuse to flourish, or to secrete their highly stimulant and aromatic properties, except in the elevated temperature and uniform moisture of tropical countries. These might have been obtained from a very broad belt, but Africa was as inaccessible, and the transit of its produce as difficult in ancient as in modern times. Asia, therefore, especially India and its islands, must always have contributed a great proportion of those articles which we now know can only be produced in tropical climates. One general observation may, I think, be applied to the whole; which is, that a large number of the more powerful drugs are produced on mountains, or in their vicinity; these affording at their bases umbrageous shelter, uniform moisture, and equable temperature, for such as require them; while the rarefied atmosphere of their sides and tops allows a free transmission of light and of heat, and, in proportion to its increased capacity for moisture, favours evaporation and the ready secretion of vegetable juices.

The History of Materia Medica, upon which I would now wish to make a few observations, is necessarily very complicated, if we attempt to study it with respect to each particular drug; for many of these have been so long used, and described by a variety of authors, in so many languages, that it is sometimes difficult for any one, without particular training, to be able to recognise the most familiar articles: I will therefore briefly relate how I was led to the study, and what means I have taken to ensure some degree of certainty in my conclusions.

Having studied the first elements of my profession under Mr., now Dr. A. T. Thomson, Professor of Materia Medica in University College, whose zeal in acquiring I ever found equalled only by his desire to communicate information; and having subsequently attended the comprehensive Course of Lectures on Materia Medica, Therapeutics, and Dietetics, by Dr. Home, in the University of Edinburgh, it may be presumed that I acquired some predilection for this branch of study. But it was only at the request of the Medical Board of Bengal, to investigate the Materia Medica of India, that I was induced to turn my attention more particularly to the subject. It would be tedious to relate the various measures I adopted for acquiring a knowledge of the substances at present in use in the several parts of that extensive empire; as well as for pointing out the sources whence a still greater variety might, if desirable, be obtained. It is enough to say, that I made collections of every thing that was procurable in their bazars, tracing them as much as possible to the plants, animals, and countries, whence they were derived. I had the native works on Materia Medica collated by competent Hakeems and Moonshees, and the several articles arranged under the three heads of the animal, vegetable, and mineral kingdoms. I made then a catalogue of the whole, in which, after the most usually received name, the several synonyms were added; and the part of the animal or plant used, the medical properties ascribed to it, and the country whence it was procured, were severally inserted. When successful in tracing the substance, I inserted the systematic Natural-Historical name, the Linnæan class and order, and especially the Natural Family of the plant. Subsequently the more important articles were arranged, according to the principles which they afforded; as acids, alkalis, fecula, gums, resins, oils, &c., also, according to their medical properties, as narcotics, tonics, cathartics, &c., and the plants according to the Natural families to which they belonged. This has enabled me, in observations on the nature and distribution of the Flora of the plains and mountains of Northern India,* to accompany them with remarks on the physical and medical properties of the different families of plants.

I trust I may be excused for entering into these details, as they are indispensable for proving that I took some trouble to make myself acquainted with the actual state of the Materia Medica of the East, and was thence enabled to pursue its history, and to trace individual articles, even under varying names and in different languages, from the present to the earliest times. It is by these means that I have been able to pick up one or two of the lost links in the history of the science.

I believe the object I have in view will be best effected by dividing the subject into the four heads of Persian, Arabian, Indian, and Greek Materia Medica.

In the first I include not only the works composed in Persia, but also those which were written in that language in India, as the plan and sources of information of all are the same. The period embraced by these authors is one of 400 years; the latest and most copious of them is the author of the *Mukhzun-al-Udwieh*, or Storehouse of Medicines, written as late as the year 1769, and printed at Hoogly in 1824. The best known of the Persian works is the *Ulfaz-Udwieh*, compiled by the Physician of the Emperor Shah Jehan. This is little more than a catalogue, but is valuable as giving the synonyms in Arabic, Persian, and Hindooee, in the Roman character, and from having been translated into English in 1793 by Mr. Gladwin. The most esteemed, however, of the Persian works, is that called *Toohft-ul Moomineen*, written in the year 1669, by Meer Mohummud Moomin, an inhabitant of Tinkaboon, in the

* Illustrations of the Botany and other branches of the Natural History of the Himalayan Mountains, and of the Flora of Cashmere.

province of Mazenderan, on the S.W. coast of the Caspian Sea. This author expressly mentions himself as the third in order of time, who had written on medicines in the Persian language, the author of the *Ikhtiarat Buddee* having been the first; and he states having completed his work in the year of the Hegira 770, which is the year 1392 of the Christian era, or 468 years from the present time, that is shortly after the close of the classic age of the School of Bagdad. Time will not permit that I should dwell at all on the contents of these works; but it is important to observe, that their several authors, in their respective Prefaces, give the dates at which they wrote, as well as the sources whence they derived their information. These they state to be their own experience, and a long list of Arabian authors, as well as translations of several Indian ones.

Passing from the Persians, we come next in the ascending series to the Arabs. They, we know, long held sway, and their works were considered of supreme authority in all the medical schools of Europe, even to the exclusion of those of the Greeks, their masters. It is needless, therefore, to refer to the merits or demerits of Avicenna, Haly Abbas, Rhazes, Serapion, or Mesue, as these are dwelt upon in the several histories of medicine. The Arabs usually receive credit for having advanced the sciences of Algebra, Astronomy, given origin to Chemistry, made some additions to Medicine, and unquestionably to our more immediate subject of Materia Medica; as many of the milder, and some of the more powerful purgatives, as well as some aromatics and stimulants, made their first appearance, as far as we at present know, in the works of Arabian authors.

The Arabian School is generally stated to have existed for 500 years. It is necessary, therefore, if we wish to connect the history of the past with the present, to ascertain by how many years the last of the Arabs preceded the first of the Persian authors, and also how soon the first of the former followed the last of the Greeks. This is the more necessary to be done, as he who closes the line, and is among the most celebrated in the East on the subject of Materia Medica, is unnoticed in our histories of medicine; probably from his works only existing in manuscript. But he was sufficiently celebrated to have attracted the notice of Gibbon, in his Decline and Fall of the Roman Empire, as well as of my late friend, Mr. Charles Mills, in his History of Muhammedanism, and has been one of the authors recommended to be translated by the Oriental Translation Committee. This is Al-Beitar, frequently called Ibn-Beitar, who flourished in the thirteenth century, and is described as having traversed Africa, Arabia, and India, in prosecution of his favourite study of Plants, particularly those yielding medicinal substances. His MSS. are preserved in the Escurial (No. 834), and are said to contain notices of several thousand plants, and to have afforded considerable assistance to the learned Bochart, in his work entitled *Geographia Sacra*, in elucidating many of the plants, animals, and precious stones, mentioned in the Bible. His works, called *Jama Ibn Beitar* and *Jama-Baghdadee*, or Collection of Ibn-Beitar and of Bagdad, are constantly quoted by the Persian authors on Materia Medica. His death is reported to have occurred in the year 1248, so as to have preceded only by 120 years the publication of the first work in the Persian language on Materia Medica.

The Arabian School being well known to have originated in the munificent patronage of the sciences by the Caliphs of Bagdad, it is necessary only to allude to the first translations from the Greek authors on Philosophy, Mathematics, Astronomy, and Medicine, having been made about A.D. 745, or just five hundred years before the death of Ibn Beitar, during the Caliphate of Al-Mansor. These translations seem first to have been made into Syriac, and afterwards into the Arabian language, by Christian Physicians of the School of Alexandria, resident at Bagdad. These Christian Physicians were held in high estimation in the Court of Harun-al-Rashid, in consequence of having cured both himself of apoplexy, and an Egyptian slave of great beauty of a dangerous illness, which had baffled the skill of the Arabian practitioners of medicine. But it was chiefly under the Caliphate of Harun's second son, Al-Mamoon, that Grecian science and medicine was made known to the Eastern World; as he, while holding the government of Khorassan, collected learned men together from all countries, and formed them into a college, appointing for their president, John Mesue of Damascus. On his father complaining that so distinguished an honour had been conferred on a Christian, Al Mamoon replied, "I have made choice of Mesue, not as a teacher of religion, but as an able preceptor in useful sciences and arts; and my father well knows, that the most learned men, and the most skilful artists in his dominions, are Jews and Christians." On succeeding to the Caliphate, Al-Mamoon employed the learned men whom he had collected in making translations of the works of Aristotle, Euclid, Ptolemy, Hippocrates, Galen, and Dioscorides. That the Arabs were still unable to proceed without the assistance of Christians, is evident from the physician Honain being the principal person employed, of whom it is related, that being threatened with death for refusing to prepare a poison, and being asked what prevented his compliance with the Caliph's command, answered, "Two things, my religion and my profession; my religion, which commands me to do good to my enemies, and my profession, which was instituted purely for the benefit of mankind."

From the Arabs we pass naturally to the Greeks, whom

they so closely followed both in time and as disciples. But it is requisite to distinguish those of the Greek authors, as *Actuarius* and *Myrepsus*, who wrote in the twelfth and thirteenth centuries, and were therefore subsequent to the chief of the Arabs; to whom it would not be difficult to prove they are largely indebted for their improved Materia Medica and Pharmacy. From these we ascend readily to Paulus Ægineta, who wrote at the beginning of the seventh century, and thence to Alexander Trallianus in the sixth, Ætius in the fifth, and from him to Oribasius, who wrote in the fourth century. Many of these are usually despised as being mere compilers; but besides the actual additions that some of them made to the science, the production of their works before the invention of printing must have been positively useful in more extensively diffusing the science of their more able predecessors. But as studying Materia Medica, and anxious to trace the history of a drug from recent to ancient times, or *vice versa*, we shall not complain of their compilations, except when they are imperfect, since they but serve to connect more closely the several links of the chain of authors, which extends from ancient to modern times.

Glancing for an instant at the continued existence of the Alexandrian School, from the times of Erasistratus and Herophilus, 300 years before the Christian era, to that of the Arabs, as accounting for the frequent appearance of Egyptian remedies among the articles of Materia Medica: we should next trace the Greek authors from Oribasius to Galen in the second century, and from him to Dioscorides, the most copious author on the Materia Medica of the ancients. He probably lived in the first century, as he is frequently quoted by Galen, and may therefore have been a contemporary of Pliny; from whom, as well as Celsus, we obtain a knowledge of the Materia Medica and Pharmacy of the Romans. Prior to Dioscorides, we have only Theophrastus, who, having died 284 years before the Christian era, gives us, in his works on Plants and Minerals, some of the earliest accounts of two of the kingdoms of nature, as Aristotle, who shortly preceded him, does of the third. This age is subsequent only by a century to that of the "Father of Medicine," whose Materia Medica can, I believe, be best ascertained, by first identifying that of his successors.

In this long enumeration of authors, who, in conjunction with medicine, have treated also of Materia Medica, the chain of connexion is upon the whole so complete, that I have found it impossible to fix upon an appropriate place for treating of the Hindoo Materia Medica authors; as these, like the writers on every other subject among this extraordinary people, are without any other than their fabulous chronology by which we may even approximatively ascertain the age in which they lived. We have, however, seen that the Persian authors at present in use in India, acknowledge having derived their information both from Indian and Arabian sources; and the latter we know have copied or appropriated what they possessed in translation from the Greeks. The Persian Materia Medica, we shall not, therefore, be surprised at finding is one of the most copious; as it is one of the most valuable, for tracing the history of the several drugs which have been in use in the Old World, from the most ancient to the present times: of these many still form some of the most important articles of our Materia Medica. Having, in the course of my investigations, referred what I found described as much as possible to both their Greek and Arabian originals, I have been able to form almost a complete circle of reference from one to the other, and thus, in a great measure, to ascertain what was original and what was copied in each.

Though the literature of his profession should never be a matter of indifference to any of its members, yet, as it was in the performance of a public duty, and not from any blind devotion to the dictates of antiquity, or especial love for the science of weighing words, that I was led to these investigations, so I endeavoured to identify the things I found named and described. The results would fill a volume, as may be seen by the MSS. on the table: the specimens which illustrate them are in the Museum. I can here adduce only a few instances to shew the nature of the information which has been, and may still be obtained, by perseverance in such inquiries.

The more common and well-known products of the East, noticed in ancient authors, it is unnecessary to mention; but there are others, which are equally described as the produce of India, but which have remained in uncertainty, or entirely undetermined. Of these, the *Lycium indicum* (λυκιον Ινδικον, Diosc.) may be given as an instance: this I found to be the extract, called *rusot*, of species of *Berberis* (*B. Lycium*, nob. and others), in use in India at the present day, as in ancient times; to this the name *lūfyon* (لوفين) is applied as the Greek term; which differs from *lūkyon* (لوقين) or λυκιον only by a diacritical point. To *Cassia Absus* the name *akakalis* (ακακαλις, Diosc. 1. c. 119) is applied: and the seed of *Cæsalpinia Bonduc* is given as one of the kinds of Eagle Stone or Ætites of the Ancients. Lupin Seeds may be obtained in the bazars of India in the present day under the name of *toormus*, evidently a corruption of θερμος. The leaves of *Cinnamomum albiflorum* and *Tammala*, which are analogous to the Bay-leaf of Europe, have *malatroon* assigned as a Greek name; apparently a corruption of *Malabathrum*. The Hemp (*Cannabis sativa*) though probably originally an Asiatic plant, has *kinnabus*, as well as *dephrunus*, assigned as its Greek, and *kinnub* as its Arabic names. In the latter language it has, in addition, a variety of other names derived from its intoxicating properties, as "increaser of pleasure,"—"cementer of friendship,"—"exciter of desire,"—"leaf of delusion," &c. Hence it has by some been thought to be the so-much-disputed *Nepenthes* of Homer. The *Acorus Calamus* (ακορος, Diosc.) sometimes called the only aromatic of European countries, is equally common in many parts of India, and has in Persian works *akoron* given as its Greek appellation.

As Dioscorides has three kinds of Nard, the Celtic, Mountain, and that which is simply called ναρδος, including the two varieties of Syrian and Indian; so, in Persian works derived from the Arabic, we have *Sunbul* or *Narden ukletee; Sunbul jibullee* (*i.e.* mountain); and *Sunbul-hindee* or Indian Nard. For this the synonymes given are, Greek, *Narden;* Latin, *Nardum;* Arabic, *Sunbul-al-teeb*, or fragrant Nard; and, Hindee, *Balchur* and *Jatamasee.* The latter is the Sanscrit, and the former the common Hindoostanee name; but under both names I obtained the hairy spike-like roots of *Nardostachys Jatamansi.* With this has often been confounded another far-famed aromatic of Eastern climes, that is, the true *Calamus aromaticus*, καλαμος αρωματικος of Dioscorides, said by him to grow in India. This he describes immediately after σχινος, which is translated *Odoratus juncus*, a produce of Africa and Arabia, and generally acknowledged by botanists to be *Andropogon Schœnanthus*, or Lemon-grass, a native both of Arabia and India, perhaps of Africa. The *Calamus aromaticus* immediately following this, stated to be also a native of India, and among other uses being mixed with ointments on account of its odour; appears to me to have been a plant allied to the former. Mentzel (Ind. Nom. Plant. Multilinguis) gives καλαμος σχοινος as one of its synonymes. It is thought also to be "the sweet cane," and "the rich aromatic reed from a far country," of Scripture; where it is spoken of as costly, and as applied to sacred uses. There is no plant which more closely coincides with every thing that is required; that is, correspondence in description; analogy to Σχινος; the possession of remarkable fragrance and stimulant properties; being costly and the produce of a far country; than the plant which yields the fragrant grass-oil of Namur (Cal. Med. Trans. vol. 1. p. 367). This oil has been already described by Mr. Hatchett, (On the Spikenard of the Ancients), who refers it to *Andropogon Iwarancusa*. It is derived, however, as appears by specimens in my possession, from a different plant; to which, believing it to be a new species, I have given the name of *Andropogon Calamus Aromaticus*.

It has frequently excited surprise, that the Arabs, so long a nation of warriors, and warriors hostile to literature, should so rapidly have become both the patrons and cultivators of science. Study of the originals, however, soon revealed that the light with which they so long shone, was borrowed from a Western source. But it was to be expected, that any people of the East would display some scintillations of genius, even though lighting their torches at the declining sun of Grecian science, as they had lent some of the earliest rays to assist its early rising. And accordingly we find that the Arabs have received credit for advancing several of the sciences, as well as that which is to be the object of our studies.

Knowing, as we now do, the laws which regulate the Geographical distribution of plants, and how much some families are confined to particular latitudes and climates; we cannot but observe, in examining the accessions made to Materia Medica by the Arabs of Bagdad, that many of the separate substances now known to be the produce of

India, or the Tropical Islands, are those for which Araby the Happy so long received the credit, as well as the affix to its name. These tropical productions could therefore be known to northern nations by the means of commerce only, or by the medium of travellers to or from those distant regions.

Since it was not the custom in those days, as now, to explore unknown or uninhabited countries, for the purpose of investigating their products, their becoming articles of commerce, or the subjects of communication to distant countries, presupposes an investigation of their properties by a resident people, willing and able to originate such inquiries. That India was peopled at a very early period, we have the concurring testimony of every ancient history: that its inhabitants were refined and intellectual, we have proofs in the sublimity of some of their early hymns, the truth and beauty of much of their poetry, the subtlety of their philosophers, and their advances in science; all evincing the conjunction of powers of observation with those of generalisation. We cannot, therefore, suppose that among so observant a people, medicine was unstudied, or the means of alleviating disease undiscovered. Accordingly, we find that these subjects were far from being neglected, and that works were written, which are still in existence, on such subjects; though it is difficult, if not impossible, to assign the age at which they were composed. From the statement of Professor Wilson, to which I shall immediately have occasion more particularly to refer, we learn that, the work ascribed to *Charak* is the most ancient, but the *Susruta*, which ranks the second in antiquity, is decidedly the first in merit.

That the Arabs were familiar with many of the products of India, is sufficiently well known, but that they were ever acquainted with any of its authors on medicine, I have never seen stated; though I hope to be able to prove the fact. I will not, for this purpose, select their descriptions of either the Cocoa or Betel-nut; Mace, Nutmeg, Tamarind, Cloves, or Cinnamon; Agallochum, that is Agila or Eagle- and Sandal-woods; Ginger, Cardamoms, or the different kinds of Pepper: nor even such medicinal articles as *Semecarpus Anacardium; Ipomæa cærulea,* called *granum indicum;* or *dund,* the *Croton Tiglium;* nor what would of itself be sufficient to prove that the Arabs had some other means than commerce, of acquiring a knowledge of Indian Materia Medica, though one of those which first roused my own attention to the subject: I mean the *Deodar, Pinus Deodara,* considered a discovery of modern times, but which is described by Avicenna under its Sanscrit name: where he says that *deiudar,* "est ex genere abhel (juniperus), que dicitur pinus Inda; et syr diudar est ejus lac," that is, turpentine. As this tree grows at considerable elevations in the interior of the Himalaya, it could only have been known to the Arabs through Hindoos, or their works.

Instead of these I take the instance which has already been adduced by Dr. Friend, to prove that the later Greek authors, as Actuarius and Myrepsus, had access to some of the Arab works; namely, the different kinds of Myrobalans, of which Dr. F. observes: "What Actuarius says of the composition of all these sorts, which is called *Tryphala,* or rather *Tryphera parva,* is exactly the same we meet with in Serapion and Mesue (whom he calls the barbarous wise men), and is recommended by them in the very same cases." (History of Medicine, 1. p. 273.) It is remarkable that not only are all the constituents of this preparation products of India, but the name of the compound itself is Sanscrit, and Sanscrit not only in use in ancient, but also in present times. Thus the three kinds of Myrobalans alluded to, the black, yellow, and Chebulic, are the produce of *Terminalia Chebula;* while the fourth, or Behera, is that of *T. Bellerica*, all belonging to the tropical family of *Combretaceæ*. The fifth, or Emblic Myrobalans, is the fruit of *Phyllanthus Emblica*, now *Emblica officinalis*, which is equally Indian. That the name *Triphala* is in use in India at present, may be seen in Shakespeare's Hindoostanee Dictionary, where the word *tirphala* is marked as Sanscrit, and explained as the name of a medicine, composed of the three *Myrobalans*. That it was similarly used in former times, may be seen in the *Amera-Cosha*, a Sanscrit Dictionary, considered as having been composed at the beginning of the Christian era; and also in Professor Wilson's paper on Leprosy, as known to the Hindoos, in the first volume of the Transactions of the Medical Society of Calcutta, p. 38, where a prescription is given from Susruta, of which *Triphala* forms one of the ingredients, and is translated as the *Three Myrobalans*.

This evidence might almost be considered sufficient to prove my point: but on referring to a translation of one of the earliest of the Arab authors, that is, Serapion, I find, under the head *De Mirobalanis*, the earliest of the Hindoo physicians, Charak, actually referred to by name. But as there is no *che* in Arabic, we have a slight change in the name, (in the same way as the Sanscrit *mocha* was converted by the Arabs into *mox*, whence our *Musa sapientum*, or *mocha* of the Brachmans), as "Et *Xarch indus* dixit in mirobalanis universaliter mirobalani sunt calidi et stiptici, et expellunt stercora ventris, et corroborant sensus omnes, et memoriam, et sensum, et conferunt lepre; et colice, et emoroidibus antiquis, et soda et ydropisi; et inducunt nauseam et vomitum:" and, again, under the head *De emblicis et belliricis*, that these, according to "*Xarcha indus* calefaciunt et sunt domini medicinarum." In Avicenna, *sub emblico*, we have a similar reference, but the name differently written, as "apud *Scirak indum*." So, in

Rhazes, who was prior to Avicenna, we have in the article De Emblico, "*Inquit Scarao indianus;*" and in that De Zingibere, "*Dixit Sarac.*" But in the article De Allio, another Indian author is quoted, whom I have not been able yet to trace out—"*Ait Sindifar* (in another place written "*Dixit Sindichar*") *indianus* valet contra ventositatem."

The Arabs were not, however, always satisfied with merely referring to the opinions of these Indian authors, but as they frequently copied from the Greeks, so have they sometimes condescended to borrow from the Hindoos. To illustrate this, I select a subject from the animal kingdom, but still confining myself to the class of remedies. Professor Wilson, in his notice respecting the medical and surgical sciences of the Hindoos, published in the Oriental Magazine, to be immediately more particularly referred to, says, "Much pains, and perhaps to but little good purpose, were bestowed upon the subject of leeches. It is said that there are twelve sorts, of which six are venomous; they are thus enumerated:—The six poisonous leeches are, the *krishna*, or black and two-headed; the *karbura*, the large-bellied leech, with a scaly hide; the *alagarda*, the hairy leech; the *indrayudha*, which is variegated like a rainbow, whence its name; the *samudrika*, which is striped yellow and black; and the *gobandana*. The bites of these produce excessive irritation, great itching, heat, and pain, spasms, sickness and syncope; and that of the *indrayudha*, even death." On referring to the chapter of Avicenna, "De Sanguisugis," and considering the double translation that the original has undergone, the coincidence is remarkable; for Avicenna says, "*Indi dixerunt* quod in quarundam sanguisugarum natura existit venenositas: ab eis igitur cavendum est, quæ sunt ex genere magna habentium capita, et quarum colores sunt antimoniales et nigræ: aut quarum color est viridis:

aut quæ sunt lanuginem habentes et similes (marmaheigi) et super quas existunt fila coloris lazuli: et quarum color similatur (almebacalbum). This is translated "iridi" in the margin, where Rhazes is referred to; "quasi omnia excepta sunt": he therefore must also have been acquainted, as indeed we have already seen was the case, with the Hindoo authors on Medicine.

Though not unwilling, because I believe it leads to truth, to pluck a few more plumes from those who heated their baths with the library of Alexandria, and littered their horses with leaves from the books of Bokhara, I feel I must not wander into other subjects, though I may touch upon one which is connected with our own. Having proved that the Arabs had access to some parts of these two Hindoo works, we are entitled to conclude that they had so to all, and to infer that as in the cases we have cited, so would they be likely to be indebted for any other new information which these contained. But this will deprive them of the honour of originating a branch of science which has always been allowed them, though I do not know that they have ever claimed it themselves; indeed, Geber, their earliest Chemist, expressly states, that he acquired his science from ancient sages.* That the Hindoos were among these, I think we may safely conclude, as Professor Wilson informs us, that the seventh division of the Ayur Veda (a work from which the above quotations were taken), is "*Rasayana*, or Chemistry, or, more correctly, Alchemy; as the chief end of the chemical combinations it describes, and which are mostly metallurgic, is the discovery of the universal medicine—the elixir that was to render health permanent, and life perpetual." But as no Hindoo work

* Totam nostram metallorum transmutandorum scientiam, quam ex libris antiquorum philosophorum abbreviamus, compilatione diversa, in nostris voluminibus, hic in unam summa redigimus.—Geber Alch. cap. 1.

on this subject has yet been translated, I am unable at present to prove directly, how much he was indebted to Hindoo authorities. Of these, the subject is the same, and treated of in the works which, as we have seen, were known to Arab authors; the style, also, as I am informed by Professor Wilson, is exactly the same, and enigmatical, like that of the old alchemists; thus similar to the well-known passage of "Bring me the six lepers that I may cleanse them;" there occurs in these ancient works of the Hindoos, "Bring me the cow that I may take off its skin."

From other sources, however, we know, that the Hindoos have long been acquainted with many chemical substances, as well as that they have practised many chemical arts. Looking to the different substances which were known to the Arabs, and some of which they are supposed first to have made known, and taking chiefly as our guide, Dr. Thomson's History of Chemistry, and the chapter entitled Chemistry of the Arabians, we shall find reason, I think, to conclude, that many of these substances must have been previously well known to the Hindoos: as common and rock salt; the former evaporated, as now, from sea-water, in the Bay of Bengal; the latter abundant in the salt rocks of the Punjab. Borax was probably obtained in former times, as at the present day from Tibet. Saltpetre must long before the time of the Arabs have been washed out of the soil, as it is in the present day, and was required for making the fire-works, for which the Indians have long been famous. Sulphate of Soda (*k,haree muttee*), they are in the present day well acquainted with, and obtain by similar means. Alum is made in Cutch, from an alum earth; it is in constant use by the Hindoos in a variety of arts as well as in medicine; and its Sanscrit name, *Phitkara*, begins with a letter which is wanting in the Arabic alphabet. Sal Ammoniac must have been familiar to the Hindoos, ever since they have burnt bricks, as they now do, with the manure of animals; as some may usually be found crystallized at the unburnt extremity of the kiln. The Egyptians obtained it from the soot of the same kind of fuel: the Sanscrit name *Nuosadur* is that, moreover, under which it is described by Arabian authors. Lime they have long known how to obtain, by burning not only limestone, but also shells and corals. Charcoal and Sulphur they were early acquainted with: the former they obtain from a variety of plants, and value that of each, according to the purposes for which it is required. Hence the Hindoos must have had the chief means for preparing many chemical products.

The alkalies even must have been known to the Hindoos: as salts from the ashes of several vegetables, and caustics made from them, are mentioned in the works to which the Arabs had access. The ashes of *Musa sapientum* and of *Butea frondosa*, most frequently mentioned for medicinal purposes, must have afforded them a carbonate of Potash; while the incineration of the Salsolas and Salicornias on the coasts of the Peninsula, and the shores of the salt lakes of North-western India, must in former, as in the present days, have afforded them a Carbonate of Soda; which is also found effloresced on the soil in some parts of their country.

The Sanscrit name of this substance being *sajika*, and the common Hindee ones *sajji muttee* and *sajji loon*, that is, sajji-earth and sajji-salt, it is remarkable that it should be described in Geber by the name of *sagimen vitri*. The latter evidently refers to its use in glass-making, an art long known to the Hindoos; and *sagimen* is a corrupted form of *sajjiloon* or *sajjinoon*; salt of *sajji*, which may be the original of *sosa* and *soda*, as *k,har* and *k,hari* may be of *kali*. Geber having been acquainted with the method of rendering these carbonates caustic by means of quicklime; it is more than probable that the Hindoos were not ignorant of the process, as directions are given in their writings for obviating the effects, when too powerful, of the caustics made from these salts. From Dr. Ainslie, we learn that a formula is contained in their works (of the date of which I am ignorant) for making ammonia, which the Tamools call *navachara acranum*, and the Dukhunees سونگنه *soongneh*, evidently derived from *soongna*, to smell. Dr. Ainslie informs us, that it is prescribed only as a local stimulant to the nose, in languors, fainting fits, and hysterics.*

The acids, also, which Geber has noticed, are found in Hindoo works, though I am unacquainted with the dates when these were written; but the differences in the processes indicate independence of investigation, if not of origin. Vinegar was known in very ancient times; but Sulphuric acid, which Geber obtained by distilling alum with a strong heat; the Tamool Vytians (physicians) prepare by burning sulphur with a small portion of nitre, in strong earthen vessels, and call *Gunduk ka atter*, essence of sulphur. Nitric acid, which Geber called *dissolving water*, and made by putting into an alembic lbj of sulphate of iron of Cyprus, ½lb. of saltpetre, and ¼lb. of alum of Jumani (Yemeni?), the Hindoos prepare by mixing together saltpetre, alum, and a portion of the liquor wrung out of cloths, spread over plants of *Cicer arietinum* (the chick pea or common gram of India). When the cloths become moistened by the deposition of dew, they more readily absorb the acid (or acidulous salt), which the plants secrete so abundantly on the surface of their leaves and shoots, and which

* The process adopted by the Hindoos, as given by Dr. Ainslie (Mat. Med. of India, I. p. 367) for making ammonia, is the following:—Take of navacharum (sal ammoniac) one pollum, simie chunamboo (chalk) two pollums; dry the two ingredients carefully, then mix them and sublime with a strong heat.

was ascertained by Vauquelin to consist of oxalic and acetic acids: the former may be useful in decomposing the nitrate of lime which is so frequently mixed with nitrate of potass. Nitro-muriatic acid, which the Arabs made by acting on sal ammoniac with nitric acid, and which they employed in dissolving gold, and called aqua regia, I have seen no notice of in the portions translated from Hindoo works; but this is probably contained in the chapter of Susruta, describing the metallurgic arts for making the elixir of life. But Muriatic acid, which Dr. Thomson does not mention as included in Geber's work, the Hindoos make by mixing together common salt and alum, previously well dried and pounded; they then add some of the above-mentioned acid liquor of the *Cicer arietinum*, and distil until the whole of the muriatic acid is disengaged and condensed in the receiver.

The metals, or at least those known to all the civilized nations of antiquity, were also known to the Hindoos, as well as to the Arabs, and gold, silver, copper, iron, lead, tin, and mercury, are mentioned in the *Amera Cosha*. But in strictly medical works, we have also notices of antimony and of arsenic, with indications of their knowledge of the ores of zinc. Indeed, one Sanscrit work is mentioned, *Rasarutna Samoochayem*, which treats of the medicines prepared with quicksilver, arsenic, and nine other metals (*Ainsl. Mat. Med.* II. p. 494); and though we have no notice of their dissolving these in the acids with which they were acquainted, this may, perhaps, be owing to those parts of their works not having yet been translated. But the oxides of several metals, as of copper, iron, lead, tin, and zinc, they were well acquainted with, and used medicinally: of lead, we find mention of both the red oxide and of litharge. With the sulphurets of iron, copper, antimony, mercury, and arsenic, both realgar and orpiment, they have long been familiar. Among the salts of the metals, we find the sulphates of copper, of zinc, and of iron, and of the latter, the red distinguished from the green: the diacetate of copper, and the carbonates of lead and of iron, are not only mentioned in their works, but used medicinally. If we had time, we might shew that some of the names by which these articles are indicated are of Hindoo origin; as *Tutia*, which occurs in Geber, but is not explained by Dr. Thomson; and *Misy*, which is mentioned by both Greek and Arabian authors.

That the substances indicated in these ancient works, were actually such as what we now understand by the English names we have assigned, is proved, as well by the names under which we can, and I have procured them in the bazars of India, as by the processes which are given for making them. So that it was not merely because some were found within the limits of their territory, that the Hindoos became acquainted with these substances; which, though a strong argument to show that they must have been acquainted with a substance, before it could have been exported to foreign countries; yet would have proved little towards their originating, or at least cultivating, chemistry prior to the Arabs, if we had not had some chemical processes to which we could confidently point. Thus, as in the case of the acids and alkalies, we here see the formation of oxides, in the directions for making the oxide of zinc; of a sulphuret, in those of mercury or factitious cinnabar; and still more interesting are the processes for making a kind of calomel, as well as of corrosive sublimate. In these a sulphuret is first formed by mixing quicksilver with fused sulphur; a layer of the black powder, which is thus obtained, is then placed over another of common salt, in a vessel half filled with small bricks; over this another vessel is directed to be luted. These are to be then placed over a strong fire for twelve hours; when cool, the muriates will be found in the uppermost. (*Ainslie* and *Fleming*.)

As the above substances are all noticed and described in medical works, we may conclude that they were so only for medical purposes. Though the ancient Greeks and Romans used many metallic substances as external applications, it is generally supposed that the Arabs were the first to prescribe them internally. Le Clerc, indeed, says, that the first physicians in Europe, who used mercury, lived in the fifteenth century, and were induced to do so from reading the works of Mesue. But in the works of Charak and Susruta, to which, as has been proved, the earliest of the Arabs had access, we find numerous metallic substances directed to be given internally; as oxide of iron, with ginger and cinnamon as a tonic; the rust in cachexy, and the sulphate in dropsy. Arsenic they prescribed not only in leprosy, and probably other cutaneous affections, but the oxide (arsenious acid) has long been with them a favourite and most efficacious remedy, in conjunction with pepper and aromatics, for the cure of intermittent fevers. Mercury appears to have been externally employed in the time of Pliny, as in his work occurs the remarkable passage (lib. xxxiii. cap. 8): "Omnia quæ de minio in medicinæ usu traduntur, temeraria arbitror: præterquam fortassis illito capite ventreve sanguinem sistendum, dum ne quid penetret in viscera, ac vulnus attingat: aliter utendum non equidem censeam." But the Hindoos have from very early times been in the habit of prescribing the sulphuret in the form of fumigation; and the preparations which we consider equivalent to calomel and to corrosive sublimate, in the form of pills combined with sugar, pepper, and aromatics; in a great variety of affections and to the extent of exciting salivation.

From the positive directions respecting the formation of these several substances, we see that the Hindoos must have been acquainted with several chemical processes, as solution and evaporation, calcination and sublimation. Distillation they have for ages practised. Mr. Hatchett, referring to Mr. Kier's paper on the method of distillation, as employed by the natives of Chatra, in Ramgur, and which is exactly the same as practised all over India; has already observed, that the antiquity and generality of the practice, and the rude simplicity of the contrivance, stamp the originality of the invention, and tend to confirm the claim of the people of India to the discovery of the art of distillation. Simple as is their apparatus, they distil with it two of the most fragrant of essences, the atur of roses, and the oil of sweet calamus, or fragrant grass-oil of Namur. That the Hindoos also practise *distillatio per descensum*, may be seen in their mode of preparing the empyreumatic oil, called *oleum nigrum*, from the seeds of *Celastrus nutans* (malkungnee), described in Mr. Malcolmson's able Prize Essay on the History and Treatment of Beriberi; which he and others found the most efficacious remedy in that intractable complaint.

Independent, however, of notices in their medical works, of the knowledge which the Hindoos possessed of many chemical processes; we might have inferred that they must have been acquainted with some, at least; from the high antiquity among them of many chemical arts, such as bleaching, dyeing, calico-printing, tanning, soap, and glass-making. The invention of gunpowder and of fireworks has often been assigned them. Working in metals they have long been famous for: their steel acquired so great celebrity at an early period, as to have passed into a proverb among the Persians, where *fouladee hind* indicates steel of the best quality; and *juwabee hind*, an Indian answer, means a cut with a sword made of Indian steel. Their works in copper and brass early attained perfection, and many of their nicer manufactures in gold and silver still continue to be admired for delicacy and beauty. This may, perhaps, be ascribed to that fineness of touch, which enabled them, in remote antiquity, to weave cottons and muslins of such unrivalled delicacy of texture, as to be sought for to clothe the kings and priests of Egypt, as well as those of the Holy Land.

Being satisfied of the existence of these Sanscrit medical works, at a period antecedent to the Arabs, it would no doubt be interesting to know something more of their contents. But no complete work, and few passages, have yet been translated into any European language. Owing, however, to the exertions of a gentleman, with whom I am proud to have been associated in the same service, who was long President of the Medical Society of Calcutta, and is now Professor of Sanscrit in the University of Oxford,—I need hardly add the name of Horace Hayman Wilson,—we are able to get a glimpse of the contents of the works of Charak and of Susruta. (v. *Calc. Orient. Magaz.* 1823; and *On Leprosy, as known to the Hindoos, Calc. Med. Trans.* vol. i.) The antiquity of the Sanscrit language is now well known, and Oriental scholars have shown its "affinity with many ancient and modern languages of Europe and Western Asia, as the Zend, the Greek and Latin, the Sclavonic, and Germanic languages." Of the estimation in which these medical works were held in other than the northern provinces of India, we have the proofs in the care and frequency with which they were translated into the languages of those parts, as Tamul on one hand, and the Tibetan on the other. The former is described as "entirely distinct, and occupying nearly as conspicuous a rank among the languages of the Peninsula, as the Sanscrit does among those of the northern provinces, as from it have been derived the Teloogoo, Malayalan, and Canarese languages." This it is necessary to know, in order to appreciate the value of the few translations which we possess of Medical works from the Tamul; as the first section of the Kalpastanum, which is a kind of compendium of the general rules of Pharmacy; and an abstract of another Indian Treatise of Medicine, published by Dr. Heyne, in his Tracts on India, p. 125-171, where he states that "most Hindoo works of any note have been originally written in Sanscrit, from which they have been translated into the modern dialects, as Tamul, Telinga," &c. A few passages have also been published by Dr. Ainslie, in his Materia Medica of India, from the works of the Megha Reesha, or Saint Aghastier or Agastya, who is usually considered as the representative of the introduction of Sanscrit Literature into the Peninsula of India, and who must be of considerable antiquity, as "he is named in the Ramayana, the oldest work most probably in the profane literature of the Hindoos" (Wilson). In addition to these, we have lately had published in English (Journ. Asiat. Soc. of Calcutta, iv. p. 1), by the celebrated Hungarian traveller, Csoma de Koros, a Synopsis of a Tibetan work on Medicine, of which the contents, he informs us, like that of the whole of Tibetan literature, has been derived from Sanscrit in the eighth century.

From such sources, I find that the Hindoos, like ancient, as well as modern practitioners every where except in large towns, practised all branches of the profession. In their works, therefore, we find notices in all departments of medicine; instances of which I have not time to adduce; but it may be sufficient to mention that, with much fanciful Anatomy, imaginative Physiology, and absurd attention to numbers, there are accounts of Poisons and their Antidotes; mention of the Diseases of Women and Children; with valuable notices relating to Surgery, Medicine, Materia Medica, and Pharmacy.

It will no doubt excite surprise, to find among the great operations of these ancient surgeons, those of Lithotomy and the extraction of the Fœtus ex utero; and that no less than 127 surgical instruments are described in their works. But I think the Professor of Surgery will agree with them when they declare, that "the first, best, and most important of all implements, is the hand," and cannot but be pleased to have his branch of the profession described, as "the first and best of the medical sciences, less liable than any other to the fallacies of conjectural and inferential practices, pure in itself, perpetual in its applicability, the worthy produce of Heaven, and certain source of fame."

With respect to Medicine, there are descriptions of the number, the origin and seat of diseases, with their symptoms, diagnosis and prognosis; accompanied, of course, with copious instructions respecting diet and treatment. Distinctions are drawn between a theoretical and practical, and observations made, as well on the character as on the duties of a Physician. Passages on the latter subjects having been translated, (one of which I owe to the kindness of Professor Wilson,) it will be seen, from his verbatim translation, that these early Hindoos had no contemptible ideas on the subject:—

"Having completed the indispensable course of study, practice is then to be as indispensably acquired; for he, who is versed in both, deserves to be honoured as the chief of physicians. As it is said (*verse*), he who is acquainted with the science of medicine only from studying the books which treat of it, and is not well grounded in the practice also, is bewildered when called upon to attend the sick, like a coward in the day of battle. He who engages in practice, presumptuously disregarding written science, is held in no estimation by the virtuous, and merits death from the King. Both these descriptions of persons are unskilful, incompetent in their profession, possessed of only one branch of the necessary qualifications, like birds with but one wing. The medicaments, which contain within them the properties of ambrosia, are as sharp weapons, the deadly thunderbolt, or fatal poisons when administered by the ignorant;—let no such man be trusted. He, who, imperfectly master of his profession, treats maladies which require either medicines or the knife, murders his patients—the vile practitioner! through his own cupidity, and the fault of the ruling authority. But he, who is conversant with both theory and practice, is competent to attain the object of his professional career, borne onwards like a war-chariot on two wheels through the ranks of the enemy."

With respect to Diagnosis, we are told that "the physician should attend chiefly to the following objects. 1. The heat of the body, which he must ascertain by feeling it with his hands. 2. Its colour: whether pale, yellowish, blackish, &c. 3. The speech: whether weak or loud. 4. The eyes. 5. The colour of the fæces: whether black, green, or yellow. 6. The urine and its colour. 7. The tongue. If all these are attentively examined by an experienced physician, they will soon point out the nature of the disease."—(Heyne's Tracts, p. 149.)

The Prognosis, whether favourable or unfavourable, is to be formed by attention to the following symptoms:—"Life," we are told, (p. 164) "is not in danger, when the following favourable symptoms occur:—When the patient takes medicines without aversion; when his voice remains unaltered; when during his well days his pulse is clear and perceptible; when he keeps himself cleanly while asleep;

when the hands and feet do not hang inertly from him; when the respiration is free and he does not expectorate too much phlegm; when he prostrates himself and adores his God in the morning, noon, and evening; when his taste is natural, and especially when he can distinguish between sour, bitter, and sweet. Under these favourable circumstances, we have no reason to be apprehensive of life, even if the patient should be very weak.

"Attention to the stars may likewise give us considerable information respecting the fate of our patient.

"The symptoms of death are as follows:—1. Want of sleep. 2. A constant murmuring, or unintelligible endeavours to speak. 3. Want of memory 4. Deep groaning breath. 5. Staring immoveable eyes. 6. Proneness to eat and to drink many improper things. 7. Disquietude. 8. Spasmodic contraction of the hands, feet, and extremities. 9. Failure of the sight. 10. An unsteady pulse, that turns to the right or left when the finger is put upon it. 11. An intermittent pulse. 12. When the body becomes cold, and the eyes stare round. 13. Dryness of the breast. 14. The protuberance of the veins, especially of that in the breast. 15. When the sides of the tongue, of the eyes, and of the joints become pale. 16. The swelling of the scrotum. 17. Burned, dry excrements. 18. Swelling of the feet and abdomen, especially of the navel. 19. Total costiveness. 20. Total want of appetite to eat or drink. 21. Constant coughing and yawning. 22. Extraordinary degree of thirst. 23. The sinking in of the eyes."

Their opinions respecting the character of a physician, were given many years ago in Sir W. Ainslie's Materia Medica of India, where, we are told, "He must be a person of strict veracity, and of the greatest sobriety and decorum; he ought to be thoroughly skilled in all the commentaries on the Ayurveda, and be otherwise a man of sense and benevolence; his heart must be charitable, his temper calm, and his constant study how to do good. Such a man is properly called a good physician; and such a physician ought still daily to improve his mind by an attentive perusal of scientific books.

"When a sick person expresses himself peevishly or hastily, a good physician is not thereby provoked to impatience; he is mild, yet courageous; and cherishes a cheerful hope of being able to save his patient's life: he is frank, communicative, impartial, and liberal; yet ever rigid in exacting an adherence to whatever regimen or rules he may think it necessary to enjoin.

"Should death come upon us, under the care of a person of this description, it can only be considered as inevitable fate, and not the consequence of presumptuous ignorance."

That the native practitioners have in some measure benefited by these instructions, we have the satisfaction to learn from a native authority in the Asiatic Researches. If the picture be a true one, I fear they would throw some of their European brethren into the shade; as it is stated, "that all the tracts on medicine must indeed be studied by the Vydyas (doctors), and they have often more learning, and far less pride than any of the Brahmins. They are usually poets, grammarians, rhetoricians, and moralists; and may, in fact, be esteemed the most virtuous and amiable of the Hindoos."

I regret that I have no such favourable passages to adduce in favour of the study of Materia Medica: but as the physician is unable to effect much good without the means it affords him; we have what is equally valuable, a long list of useful medicines, of which many continue to be employed in modern as in very ancient times. As we might expect from the mild habits, simple diet, and unexcitable constitutions of the Hindoos, with attention to regimen, there is a long list of what are translated assuaging and depuratory medicines. But as we should likewise expect from the observers of nature, in a country where the accession of disease is as sudden as is the rapid accumulation of fearfully fatal symptoms; which are to be arrested only by promptness of decision, and vigour of practice; so for such cases the Hindoo sages have observed the efficacy of blood-letting, cupping and leeches, with drastic and mild purgatives, emetics, diaphoretics, baths, and aspersions of water. Some of the acrid poisons even, were used at this early period, with, as we have seen, arsenic and mercurial preparations, as well as stimulants, sedatives, and narcotics. With respect to their prescriptions and works, Professor Wilson makes the valuable remark, that in proportion as the work is more modern, the compounds become more extravagant, and assume a more important place in the practice. But India, gentlemen, is not the only country where the simplicity and clearness of observers has been displaced by the obscurity and mystification of compilers.

The arrangement of Materia Medica, in the Susruta,* is one which I do not recollect to have elsewhere seen, but one portion of which plainly betrays its origin. All medicines are divided into locomotive and non-locomotive:—among the former are included all animals, whether viviparous, oviparous, or produced in moist places. On the banks of the Ganges, as on those of the Nile, we see the phenomena resulting from moisture and heat in the swarming of animal forms, gave rise to the doctrines of

* My attention was lately more particularly called to the Materia Medica of Susruta by Dr. de Glehn, from St. Petersburgh, who did me the favour of a visit to inquire into the state of medicine in India; as he had, with the assistance of Dr. Rosen, obtained some insight into the contents of that Sanscrit author.

equivocal generation. Among the non-locomotive medicines, plants are placed, and are followed by mineral medicines; among which, gold, silver, arsenic, mercury, diamonds, pearls, and earths, are enumerated. Heat and cold, light and darkness, the increase and decrease of the moon's age, are mentioned as means to be employed in the cure of diseases. Thus we see sol-lunar influence very early attracted the attention of physicians in tropical countries. In the Kalpastanum also, we are told, that "as patients are apt to grow worse in the night, double doses of medicine should be given them in the evening. These nightly exacerbations are owing to the influence of the moon, and especially of its beams, which produce injurious effects even on healthy persons."

In the last-mentioned work, medicinal drugs and plants are arranged under the following heads: Tuberous and Bulbous Roots; Roots; Bark of Roots; Bark of large Trees; Trees possessing a peculiar smell; Leaves; Flowers; Fruits; Seeds; Acrid and Astringent Vegetables; Milky Plants; Gums and Resins. This work is also extremely interesting, as giving probably the earliest notices respecting Botanical Geography; the sites and climates where different kinds of plants grow; the soils and seasons whence, and when medicinal plants should be collected; modes of keeping medicines and their preparation; time during which they remain good; with the weights and measures to be used. Among the rules of Pharmacy, we have directions for making Rasaha, or the expressed juice of fresh vegetables; Kalkaha, the powder of well-dried plants; Sitaha, cold infusions; Srutaha, Kashaim and Pandaha, decoctions. Ingredients that are added to the decoction after the boiling is over, as syrup, honey, pippaly, salts, &c. are called Brativapam by the Sastrums. Decoctions made with oil are called Tailam.

Some authors, it is said, prescribe decoctions made of meat. The Leham or electuary, is composed of a strong decoction of dry powdered ingredients, and some oil, or ghee (clarified butter), and sugar or honey. Dr. Heyne also gives, from the Treatise on Medicine, the directions for making "Flowers of Zinc," also of their "Iron Cendurams," which are "so many modes of preparing martial ethiops," informing us that they "consider the colour of medicines prepared from metals, as the greatest criterion of their excellence." There are also several preparations of copper, which the Hindoos have long used both internally and externally. In the midst of the good sense displayed in many of their practical instructions, we may in these days smile at the ceremonies with which these are directed to be accompanied. Thus it is explained, "that by the prayers and reading of the Veda by the Bramins, Brahma and Vishnu will be pleased; by the light we conciliate the favour of Bhagavatadu, or the supreme being; by the heaps of the different kinds of grain we please the nine heavenly bodies; by the painted ground in particular we gratify the sun; by the painted goblet, Aswāry, the god of physic; and by the pearls and precious stones we conciliate the favour of Latchmy Davie, the goddess of riches."—(p. 147.)

And it is further recommended for his good, that "Before the patient takes the medicine, the god of physic is to be worshipped, in the person of his deputy, the physician, who must be paid well for his services."

In the abstract of the Tibetan work, all medicines are subdivided as remedial agents, into thirty-seven different classes, and consist of 715 different substances. With respect to such as I am acquainted with, in all these old works, it appears to me, that with the exception of Assafœtida, mentioned in the *Amera-Cosha*, I can see none but what are indigenous in India.*

The foregoing extracts, together with those in the sub-

* As the work (Oriental Magazine, Calcutta, February and March 1823) in which the notices respecting early Hindoo medicines were anonymously published by Professor Wilson is not easily to be procured, except at Messrs. Allen and Co.'s, Leadenhall-street, it will not, I conceive, be out of place, to insert some extracts from these notices and translations.

Professor Wilson commences with a few preliminary observations, in which he states, "that there is reason to conclude, from the imperfect opportunities of investigation we possess, that in medicine, as in astronomy, and metaphysics, the Hindus once kept pace with the most enlightened nations of the world; and that they attained as thorough a proficiency in medicine and surgery, as any people, whose acquisitions are recorded, and as indeed was practicable, before anatomy was made known to us, by the discoveries of modern inquirers.

"It might easily be supposed, that their patient attention, and natural shrewdness, would render the Hindus excellent observers; whilst the extent, and fertility of their native country would furnish them with many valuable drugs and medicaments. Their *Nidan*, or Diagnosis, accordingly appears to define and distinguish symptoms with great accuracy, and their *Druvyabhidhana*, or Materia Medica, is sufficiently voluminous. They have also paid great attention to regimen and diet, and have a number of works on the food and general treatment, suited to the complaint, or favourable to the operation of the medicine administered. This branch they entitle *Pathapathya*. To these subjects are to be added, the *Chikitsa*, or medical treatment of diseases—on which subject they have a variety of compositions, containing much absurdity, with much that is of value; and the *Rasavidya*, or Pharmacy, in which they are most deficient."

— "The *Ayur Veda*, as the medical writings of highest antiquity and authority are collectively called, is considered to be a portion of the fourth or *Atharva Veda*, and is consequently the work of Brahma—by him it was communicated to Dacsha, the *Prajapati*, and by him, the two Aswins, or sons of Surya, the Sun, were instructed in it, and they then became the medical attendants of the gods—a genealogy, that cannot fail recalling to us the two sons of *Esculapius*, and their descent from *Apollo*. Now what were the duties of the Aswins, according to Hindu authorities?—the gods, enjoying eternal youth and health, stood in no need of physicians, and consequently these held no such sinecure station. The wars between the gods and demons, however, and the conflicts amongst the gods themselves, in which wounds might be suffered, although death was not inflicted, required chirurgical aid—and it was this, accordingly, which the two Aswins rendered.

joined notes from Hindoo works, viewed in connexion with the apparent antiquity and independent origin of their Medicine, display, I conceive, considerable merit, not only

dered. They performed many extraordinary cures, as might have been expected, from their superhuman character.

"The meaning of these legendary absurdities is clear enough, and is conformable to the tenor of all history. Man, in the semi-barbarous state, if not more subject to external injuries, than internal disease, was at least more likely to seek remedies for the former, which were obvious to his senses, than to imagine the means of relieving the latter, whose nature he could so little comprehend.

"Surgical, therefore, preceded medicinal skill; as Celsus has asserted, when commenting on Homer's account of Podalirius and Machaon, who were not consulted, he says, during the plague in the Grecian camp, although regularly employed, to extract darts and heal wounds. The same position is maintained, as we shall hereafter see, by the Hindu writers, in plain, as well as in legendary language.

"According to some authorities, the Aswins instructed Indra, and Indra was the preceptor of Dhanwantari; but others make Atreya, Bharadwaja, and Charaka, prior to the latter. Charaka's work, which goes by his name, is extant—Dhanwantari is also styled *Kasiraja*, prince of *Kasi* or Benares. His disciple was Susruta, the son of Viswamitra, and consequently a contemporary of Rama: his work also exists, and is our chief guide at present. It is unquestionably of some antiquity, but it is not easy to form any conjecture of its real date, except that it cannot have the prodigious age, which Hindu fable assigns it—it is sufficient to know, that it is perhaps the oldest work on the subject, excepting that of Charaka, which the Hindus possess. One commentary on the text, made by Ubhatta, a Cashmirian, is probably as old as the twelfth or thirteenth century, and his comment, it is believed, was preceded by others. The work is divided into six portions—the *Sutra St'hana*, or Chirurgical Definitions; the *Nidana St'hana*, or section on Symptoms, or Diagnosis; *Sarira St'hana*, anatomy; *Chikitsa St'hana*, the internal application of Medicines; *Kalpa St'hana*, Antidotes; *Uttara St'hana*, or a supplementary section on various local diseases, or affections of the eyé, ear, &c.—In all these divisions, however, surgery, and not general medicine, is the object of the *Susruta*.

"The *Ayur Veda*, which originally consisted of one hundred sections, of a thousand stanzas each, was adapted to the limited faculties and life of man, by its distribution into eight subdivisions, the enumeration of which conveys to us an accurate idea, of the objects of the *Ars medendi* amongst the Hindus. The divisions are thus enumerated—1. *Salya*; 2. *Salakya*; 3. *Kaya chikitsa*; 4. *Bhutavidya*; 5. *Kaumarabhritya*; 6. *Agada*; 7. *Rasayana*; and 8. *Bajikarana*.—They are explained as follows:

1. "*Salya*

as shewing that they had at an early period paid attention to what now constitute the several branches of medicine, but also that they had discovered the various kinds of remedies,

1. " *Salya* is the art of extracting extraneous substances, whether of grass, wood, earth, metal, bone, &c. violently or accidentally introduced into the human body; with the treatment of the inflammation and suppuration thereby induced; and by analogy, the cure of all phlegmonoid tumours and abscesses. The word *Salya* means a dart or arrow, and points clearly to the origin of this branch of Hindu science. In like manner the Ἰατρὸς, or physician of the Greeks, was derived, according to *Sextus Empiricus*, from Ἰὸς, an arrow or dart.

2. " *Salakya* is the treatment of external organic affections, or diseases of the eyes, ears, nose, &c.; it is derived from *Salaka*, which means any thin and sharp instrument; and is either applicable in the same manner as *Salya*, to the active causes of the morbid state, or it is borrowed from the generic name of the slender probes and needles, used in operations on the parts affected.

3. " *Kaya Chikitsa* is, as the name implies, the application of the Ars medendi (*Chikitsa*) to the *body* in general (*Kaya*), and forms what we mean by the Science of Medicine—the two preceding divisions constitute the Surgery of modern schools.

4. " *Bhutavidya* is the restoration of the faculties from a disorganised state, induced by Demoniacal possession. This art has vanished before the diffusion of knowledge, but it formed a very important branch of medical practice, through all the schools, Greek, Arabic, or European, and descended to days very near our own, as a reference to *Burton's* Anatomy of Melancholy may prove to general readers.

5. " *Kaumara bhritya* means, the care of infancy, comprehending not only the management of children from their birth, but the treatment of irregular lactic secretion, and puerperal disorders in mothers and nurses—this holds with us also the place, that its importance claims.

6. " *Agada* is the administration of antidotes—a subject which, as far as it rests upon scientific principles, is blended with our medicine and surgery.

7. " *Rasayana* is chemistry, or more correctly alchemy, as the chief end of the chemical combinations it describes, and which are mostly metallurgic, is the discovery of the universal medicine—the elixir, that was to render health permanent, and life perpetual.

8. " The last branch, *Bajikarana*, professes to promote the increase of the human race—an illusory research, which, as well as the preceding, is not without its parallel in ancient, and modern times.

" We have, therefore, included in these branches, all the real and fanciful pursuits of physicians of every time and place. Susruta, however, confines his own work to the classes, *Salya* and *Salakya*, or Surgery; although, by an arrangement not uncommon with our own writers, he introduces occasionally as well as the modes of applying them. That many of these are of a valuable nature, we may readily be assured by looking at their Materia Medica, or our own obli-

occasionally the treatment of general diseases, and the management of women and children, when discussing those topics, to which they bear relation."

—"The practical part of the subject of Surgery is preceded by a few general remarks. 'Living bodies are composed,' it is said, 'of the five elements, with action or life superadded: they are produced from vapour, vegetation, incubation, and parturition, as insects, plants, birds, fishes, reptiles, and animals. All the Hindu systems consider vegetable bodies, as endowed with life. Of animals, man is the chief, and in proportion to his complicated structure is his liability to disease. The disorders of the human frame are of four kinds; accidental, organic, intellectual, and natural. The injuries arising from external causes form the first class; the second comprehends the effects of the vitiated humours, or derangements of the blood, bile, wind, and phlegm; the third class is occasioned by the operation of the passions, or the effects on the constitution of rage, fear, sorrow, joy, and others; and the last is referable to the necessary, and innate condition of our being, as thirst, hunger, sleep, old age, and decay."

—"The instrumental part of medical treatment was, according to the best authorities, of eight kinds—*Chhedana*, cutting or scission; *Bhedana*, division or excision; *Lek'hana*, which means *drawing lines*, appears to be applied to scarification and inoculation; *Vyadhana*, puncturing; *Eshyam*, probing, or sounding; *Aharya*, extraction of solid bodies; *Visravana*, extraction of fluids, including venesection; and *Sevana*, or sewing: and the mechanical means, by which these operations were performed, seem to have been sufficiently numerous. Of these, the principal are the following:

"*Yantras*, properly machines, in the present case instruments; but to distinguish them from the next class, to which that title more particularly applies, we may call them implements; *Sastras*, weapons, or instruments; *Kshara*, alkaline solutions, or caustics; *Agni*, fire, the actual cautery; *Salaka*, pins, or tents; *Sringa*, horns, the horns of animals open at the extremities, and, as well as *Alabu* or gourds, used as our cupping glasses; the removal of the atmospheric pressure through the first being effected by suction, and in the second by rarifying the air by the application of a lamp. The next subsidiary means are *Jalauka*, or leeches.

"Besides these, we have thread, leaves, bandages, pledgets, heated metallic plates for erubescents, and a variety of astringent or emollient applications."

— The detailed descriptions of the very numerous Hindu instruments not being very minute or precise, Professor Wilson says, we can only conjecture what they may have been, from a consideration of the purport of gations to it; as well as by remembering how recently some among them of old date, have been introduced into European practice; as the smoking of Datura leaves in asthma;

of their names, and the objects to which they were applied, in conjunction with the imperfect description given.

"The *Sastras*, or cutting instruments, were of metal, and should be always bright, handsome, polished, and sharp, sufficiently so, indeed, to divide a hair longitudinally."

—"The means by which the young practitioner is to obtain dexterity in the use of his instruments are of a mixed character; and whilst some are striking specimens of the lame contrivances to which the want of the only effective vehicle of instruction, human dissection, compelled the Hindus to have recourse, others surprise us by their supposed incompatibility with what we have been hitherto disposed to consider as insurmountable prejudices. Thus the different kinds of scission, longitudinal, transverse, inverted, and circular, are directed to be practised on flowers, bulbs, and gourds. Incision, on skins, or bladders, filled with paste and mire;—scarification, on the *fresh hides of animals, from which the hair has not been removed;*—puncturing, or lancing, on the hollow stalks of plants, or *the vessels of dead animals;*—extraction *on the cavities of the same,* or fruits with many large seeds, as the Jack and Bel;—sutures, on skin and leather, and ligatures and bandages on well-made models of the human limbs. The employment of leather, skin, and even of dead carcases, thus enjoined, proves an exemption from notions of impurity we were little to expect, when adverting to their actual prevalence. Of course, their use implies the absence of any objections to the similar employment of human subjects; and although they are not specified, they may possibly be implicated, in the general direction which the author of the Susruta gives, that the teacher shall seek to perfect his pupil by the application of all expedients, which he may think calculated to effect his proficiency."

—"Of the supplementary articles of Hindu surgery, the first is *Kshara*, alkaline or alkalescent salts. This is obtained by burning different vegetable substances, and boiling the ashes with five or six times their measure of water. In some cases the concentrated solution is used after straining, and is administered internally, as well as applied externally."

—"Care is enjoined in their use, and emollient applications are to be applied, if the caustic occasions very great pain. At the same time these and the other substitutes for instrumental agents are only to be had recourse to, where it is necessary to humour the weakness of the patient. They are especially found serviceable, where the surgeon has to deal with princes and persons of rank, old men, women and children, and individuals of a timid and effeminate character."

—"The cautery is applied by hot seeds, combustible substances inflamed, boiling fluids of a gelatinous or mucous consistence, and heated metallic bars, the prescribing of Nux vomica in paralysis and dyspepsia, and the revival of the use of *Croton Tiglium*. From the mixture, however, of much ignorance and absurdity with what is valuable, many will be apt to despise altogether the Medicine of the East. But if it be recollected how long in Europe prevailed the influence of Galen; as well as how many absurd formulæ still figure in some continental Pharmacopœias, as also how comparatively recent is the time since our own was so greatly improved; some feeling of humiliation will control the pride with which we now view the medical sciences. As records of early civilisation, and as elucidating the history of medicine, a more

bars, plates, and probes. The application is useful in many cases, as to the temples and forehead, for head-aches; to the eye-lids, for diseases of the eyes; to the part affected, for indurations in the skin; to the sides, for spleen and liver; and to the abdomen, for mesenteric enlargements. As amongst the Greeks, however, the chief use of the cautery was in the case of hemorrhages, bleeding being stopped by searing the wounded vessels."

— "If leeches, when applied, are slow and sluggish, a little blood may be drawn from the part by a lancet, to excite their vivacity; when they fall off, the bleeding may be maintained by the use of the horns and gourds, or the substitutes already mentioned, for the cupping glasses of our own practice."

— "The operations are rude, and very imperfectly described. They were evidently bold, and must have been hazardous:—their being attempted at all is however most extraordinary, unless their obliteration from the knowledge, not to say the practice, of later times, be considered as a still more remarkable circumstance. It would be an inquiry of some interest, to trace the period and causes of the disappearance of Surgery from amongst the Hindus—it is evidently of comparatively modern occurrence, as operative and instrumental practice forms so principal a part of those writings, which are undeniably most ancient; and which, being regarded as the composition of inspired writers, are held of the highest authority."

Besides these sacred writings, there are many valuable professional tracts which correspond with, and are, in fact, commentaries on them. These are said to have been composed by prophets and holy men (Magha Reeshees), to whom is generally given a divine origin.

The different nations of India have their respective medical authors. In the Peninsula and the South of India, in Tamul; those of the Telingas in Teloogoo; in Bengal and the Northern Provinces, the works in use among the Hindoos are in Sanscrit; while among the Mahomedan population, Persian works and translations from the Arabic are chiefly in use.

intimate knowledge of the contents of these Hindoo works would be highly interesting; and I hope that there is sufficient zeal in the profession here, as well as in India, to command the translation of at least the two oldest works, (those of Charak and Susruta,) as well as of one on each of the different departments, to give European readers a complete view of Hindoo Medicine, and enable us to weigh its claims to originality.

Hindoo works on Medicine having been proved to have existed prior to the Arabs, little doubt can be entertained, I conceive, respecting their originality; as we know of no source from which they could have been borrowed, except from the Greeks; and there is little probability of the Hindoos having had access to any original or translated works at so early a period, as must have been the case from their containing no traces of the Galenical doctrines so conspicuous in the writings of the Arabs. Some coincidences would appear rather to be that of observers of the same facts, than of borrowers from the same books. The description of some diseases which seem to have been first known in India, as well as the internal administration of metals, they could not have borrowed from the Greeks. That there must have been independent observers in India, at a very early age of the world, we have proofs in the commerce of their manufactures and of their medicines. Many of the latter may be found described in the works of the Greeks, but we see no trace of European medicines in those of the Hindoos; and though knowledge may travel from north to south, tropical products can in our hemisphere only travel from south to north. Their employment, therefore, in the latter, proves their previous investigation by a people resident in the countries of their growth. On such grounds, therefore, I conceive, we may infer the antiquity of Hindoo medicine; and while unable to get any positive dates for their works, we may yet, by circumstantial evidence, obtain an approximation which will, I think, prove its independent origin. We may, however, conceive it to be the remains of a still more ancient system, of which we have no records, but of the existence of which there can be no doubt, as Herodotus relates, that in his time, in Egypt, there were distinct physicians for different diseases, which were classed according to their seat in the human body; and from Diodorus Siculus we learn, that every physician was obliged to follow a written code. Hence it is more than probable that there was early in Egypt a distinct system of medicine, and we have notices also in the works of the ancients of its being a subject much attended to by the Persian magi. Notwithstanding that the Greeks travelled to the East and to Egypt in quest of knowledge, it has been said, that Egyptian medicine consisted chiefly in incantation; but this explanation is as likely to have been owing to the ignorance of the narrators as of the physicians; for even in our own day we seldom see even well-informed writers able to explain or to describe correctly facts of a scientific nature. In the same manner, those who were unable to decypher their hieroglyphics, pronounced all the knowledge of the Egyptian priesthood to consist in magic.

The only direct testimony we have with respect to the date of the works of Charak and of Susruta, is that of Professor Wilson, who states that from their being mentioned in the Puranas, the ninth or tenth century is the most modern limit of our conjecture; while the style of the authors, as well as their having become the heroes of fable, indicate a long anterior date. The Arabs must have become acquainted with the translations in the eighth, or early in the ninth century, as Harun-al-Rashid and Al-Mamoon succeeded respectively in the years 786 and 813 to the Caliphate, when it stretched to the Indus: the latter survived only twenty years. Geber is supposed to have lived in the seventh or eighth century, and we have shewn the probability of his having had access to the chemical knowledge of the Hindoos. But for their merits to have been sufficiently established for their works to be translated at the same time with those of the principal Greek authors, these Hindoo physicians must certainly have lived and written long before; to allow their fame to extend into foreign countries, in an age when the communication of literature must have been at least as slow as it now is in the East.*

* Having mentioned to Professor Wilson the discovery I had made, of the Arabs having been indebted to the Hindoos for some of the information for which they have hitherto received credit, he informed me that he had seen a notice in the Foreign Quarterly Review, of a German physician having made the same discovery. I looked through every number of that periodical, but was unable to find the notice alluded to. It is only since the foregoing part has been in type, that Professor Wilson has informed me, that the notice was contained in the Journal of Education. On applying to Messrs. Taylor and Walter, booksellers to University College, they were good enough to look out the passage for me, where may be seen, in volume viii. p. 176, that " Dietz, one of the medical professors at the University of Königsberg, who has spent five years of his life in visiting the principal libraries of Germany, Italy, Switzerland, Spain, France, and England, in search of manuscripts of ancient Greek, Roman, and Oriental writers on Medicine, is now engaged in publishing his 'Analecta Medica.' The work contains several interesting papers on the subject of Physical Science among the Indians and Arabians, and communicates several introductory notices and illustrations from native Eastern writers. Dietz proves that the late Greek physicians were acquainted with the medical works of the Hindus, and availed themselves of their medicaments; but he more particularly shews, that the Arabians were familiar with them, and extolled the healing art, as practised by the Indians, quite as much as that in use among the Greeks. It appears from Ibn Osaibe's testimony (from whose biographical work Dietz has given a long abstract on the. Lives of Indian Physicians), that a variety of treatises on Medical Science were translated from the Sanscrit into Persian and Arabic, particularly the more important compilations of Charaka and Susruta, which are still held in estimation in India; and that Manka and Saleh, the former of whom translated a special treatise on Poison into Persian, even held appointments as body-physicians

at

If we now consider the period when translations were first made from these works into other languages, though indicating rather the age when neighbouring

at the Court of Harun-al-Rashid." The fact of the translation of numerous works on medicine from the Sanscrit into Arabic we have long known, from the list of those works given by Sir W. Ainslie at the end of his Materia Indica; but the age when these translations were made we were unacquainted with. The nature of the works of Charaka and Susruta we had a glimpse of from Professor Wilson's translations; but the fact of Manka and Saleh being at the Court of Harun-al-Rashid is extremely curious, as well as that of the later Greek physicians having had access to some Hindoo works. Actuarius and Myrepsus are unimportant, as both were subsequent to the Arabs; but even previous to them, as I have more than once mentioned to Professor Wilson, the occurrence of long prescriptions, composed of tropical products, appeared to me to be taken from Hindoo works.

The work of Susruta, it may be useful to remark, is now easily procurable, as it was one of those ordered to be printed by the Indian Government for the use of its native subjects; but strange to say, the printing was stopped, of this as well as of many others, when most were nearly completed: the first volume and three-fourths of the second of the Susruta having been printed. Fortunately the Asiatic Society of Calcutta, with the spirit and zeal which has ever distinguished it, and with a true knowledge of what was for the benefit of the government itself, undertook, at their own risk, to complete the abandoned works. If the occurrence had not been so recent, it might, like the burning of the Alexandrian library, from its incredibility, have afforded disputants or defenders an opportunity of denying, or, at least, doubting the fact. The Asiatic Society has been energetically supported in its representations by the Royal Asiatic Society; and it is gratifying to state, also by the "Société Asiatique" of Paris, and by German literati, in promoting the sale of these works on the Continent. That their efforts, coupled with the accession of Lord Auckland to the Indian Government have been in some degree successful, we have the assurance, in comparing the statement at the end of 1835 with that at the conclusion of the year 1835, of the Editor of the Journal of the Asiatic Society of Calcutta.

"Without venturing to impugn in any degree the wisdom or policy of a measure, which has in the face of all India withdrawn the countenance of government from the learned natives of the country, and pronounced a verdict of condemnation and abandonment on its literature, it may be allowable in this place to prophecy, that the conduct of the Asiatic Society, in stepping forward to rescue the half-printed volumes of Sanscrit, Arabic, and Persian, will be approved and applauded by every learned Society and every scholar in Europe. Left in their unfinished state, they would have indeed merited the opprobrious designation of an 'accumulation of waste paper,' nations were able to appreciate the value of such works than the time when they were written, we still get a confirmation of the previous testimony. Thus they were translated into Tamul by the Maha Rishi Aghastier, (v. p. 48), who appears to have introduced the religion, as well as the science of the Hindoos, into the Peninsula before the Christian era. That the Hindoos of the north had communication anterior to that date with the inhabitants of the south, has been proved by Mr. Turnour, who has been able to shew, from Pali annals, the connexion between Ceylon and Ancient Behar, from the period of the rise in the latter of Buddhism (543 B.C.) nearly six centuries before the Christian era. This connexion is attested, according to the Rev. Dr. Mill, by the very language in which these annals are written: the Pali being no other than the classical form of a peculiar modification of Sanscrit speech in Ancient Behar. The general correctness of these annals has, among other facts, been further confirmed by their containing the names of six sovereigns, whose existence had been indicated by coins only recently found in India. (Journ. As. Soc. Calcutta, v. p. 829). Sanscrit Medical Literature, we have seen, (p. 48) was introduced into Tibet in the eighth century; whence it probably spread further eastward, though we have no means of ascertaining the fact; but I think it likely that

paper,' applied to them by the government which had originally ordered, and had expended vast sums upon, their publication." (Dec. 1835).

"If, in our last volume, we could not refrain from noticing, as the most prominent object of interest in its contents, the suspension of oriental publications by the British Indian Government, and the general discouragement under which oriental studies were doomed to languish, we must not, on the present occasion, omit to make honourable mention of the patronage and favour which has once more dawned upon science and literature in India under the present administration. The proceedings of the Asiatic Society, last year so full of painful discussion and unsuccessful appeal, this year shine forth with tokens of distinguished consideration." (Dec. 1836).

some connexion will be found to have existed between the medicine of the Hindoos and that of the Chinese.

On the subject of Chinese Medicine, we have a short notice, and another on the Chinese Treatment of Paralysis, in the Calcutta Medical Transactions, Vol. I., (p. 146), where it is stated that the Science of Medicine may be said to have commenced with Chang-ke (about A.D. 229); for all works before that (said to be dated 189 and 1105 years B.C.) treat of medicine, without giving prescriptions. As this is extracted from a new compilation made by order of the Emperor in 1789, it is difficult, from the necessary changes in arrangement and the heading of chapters, to be able to trace the sources whence they may have been derived, or where they communicated information. But it may be remarked as important, that small-pox is noticed, both in this and the Tibetan work, in conjunction with infectious diseases in general. More recently, Mr. Gutzlaff, Missionary in China, has in the Proceedings of the Asiatic Society, part vii. p. 154, given a short view of a celebrated work, in forty volumes, on Chinese Medicine, which is called "Ching che chun ching," *i.e.* "Approved marking line of Medical Practice." Of this, seven volumes consist of Nosology, *Tsa-ching;* eight of Pharmacology, *Luy-fang;* five of Pathology, *Shang-han;* six of Surgery, *Wae-ka;* and the remaining volumes treat of the diseases of Women and Children. The Chinese Pharmacopœia is described as being very extensive; almost every shrub, leaf or root, being adopted as an article of Materia Medica. Among many indigenous products, of which we may get a pretty accurate idea from the drawings which have been published, as well as from the collection of Chinese Materia Medica, in the possession of the College of Physicians; there are others, which they import from foreign countries. Among the former may be mentioned musk, rhubarb, ginseng, the larvæ of the silk-worm, &c.; while among the exotic articles are opium, assafœtida, and many aromatics, as nutmegs, cloves, cinnamon, and pepper. It is curious to observe the number of animal products which they employ as medicinal articles; as the bones of tigers and elephants, the horns of animals, and the fins of fishes, with reptiles, snails, and scorpions. It is interesting to find among them also, the employment internally of cinnabar and the oxide of mercury, as well as of the oxide and sulphuret of arsenic. I may briefly remark, that many articles are common to the Hindoo and Chinese lists of Materia Medica. From the translation of a Chinese account of India, published in the Asiatic Journal, July 1836, it will be seen that there was constant intercourse between these countries even before the Christian era, by means of travellers and ambassadors; and that Buddhist priests in visiting China, took with them as presents classical Indian books. It is also worthy of notice, in connexion with the chapter on this subject in Susruta, that in A.D. 648, the Emperor of China having sent an ambassador to India, this officer met with a doctor, who told him that he was 200 years old, and that he possessed the recipe of immortality. Upon hearing which, a second embassy was dispatched in search of the philosophical stone.

If we now revert to the north, we may readily concede that from the position and history of Persia, there must always have been considerable intercourse between it and India. But independent of this, we have positive testimony on the subject, as the Baron de Sacy, in his account of the now well-known Sanscrit origin of the Fables of Pilpay, states that these were first translated into Pehlevi during the reign of the Persian King Nooshirwan, who ascended the throne in 531, and died in 579; and who is reported by historians to have encouraged learning, and to have introduced Grecian philosophy at his court. The translations were made by the Physician Barzouyeh who had brought the original from India with other books, and who by more than one previous journey to that country, had acquired a knowledge of Sanscrit. He is stated particularly, to have made two journeys, one for the purpose of procuring medicaments and herbs, and the other for obtaining specimens of the literature of the Hindoos.

That commercial intercourse subsisted between India and the Babylonians and Assyrians, is generally admitted; that in this the Persians subsequently participated, is well known, as well as that they invaded India, and held sovereignty over some of the north-western provinces. But that the Persians obtained any knowledge of the medicine of the Hindoos, when they first became acquainted with their literature, we are not informed. From a physician, however, visiting Hindoosthan to procure medicaments and books, we are assured that the former were then in high repute, and that their virtues had been described by the authors, or at least ascertained by the practitioners of medicine in India. Some therefore may have formed a portion of the trade which always subsisted between these countries, and of which Assafœtida, and perhaps some of the other fœtid gum-resins, formed a part of the return which Persia made for the spices and aromatics of the East.

That some of these did form articles of commerce in very ancient times, we know from the accounts of Greek and Roman writers; that they were employed not only as condiments, but also as medicines, we likewise know from their being included in the most ancient lists of Materia Medica, with some, as *Lycium indicum*, which could only have been employed as medicines. These might certainly have all become known to the nations of the West, through the medium of Egypt, which was early visited by Grecian Philosophers; and to which, from remote antiquity, an active commerce was carried on along the Red Sea, by the Arabs of Yemen. They, as well as the Phœnicians, may have been enabled to visit India even in the infancy of navigation, either by coasting or by the aid of the monsoons. But this commerce, long as it had been established, and extensive as it no doubt was, cannot be compared, in the opinion of Heeren, with that which had, from probably earlier times, always taken place by land.

As the Persian Court and kingdom were for nearly twelve centuries in the most flourishing condition, they necessarily became the resort of travellers and merchants from all parts of the world. Here, therefore, the products of the East must at an early time have been in great demand: and, here, as well as in Egypt, they may have become known to the philosophers and physicians of Greece. That these resorted to, and were held in high estimation at, the Court of Persia, when this held sway over some of the north-western provinces of India, is easily proved. Even as early as 430 B.C., or during the plague of Athens, with which the inhabitants of Persia were also afflicted, Artaxerxes is said to have invited Hippocrates to his Court: and though neither the proposal, nor the answer of the latter refusing to leave his countrymen at such a juncture, is credited, there can be no doubt of the high estimation in which Greek physicians were then held, as only thirty years later, Ctesias was Physician to the Persian sovereign, and remained in that capacity for seventeen years, during which he wrote a history of the Persian Empire, and an account of India, the latter of which has been shewn by Professor Wilson, in a paper read to the

Ashmolean Society of Oxford, to contain notices of the natural productions of the country, which, though often extravagant and absurd, are nevertheles founded on truth. Besides, there were always Grecian mercenaries in Persian pay; and the Grecian prisoners taken at Eretria were settled in Persia, within a day's journey of Susa. In the year 330 B.C., Darius Codomanus was killed, and an end put to the Kaianian dynasty of the Persian empire by Alexander, who carried his arms to the shores of the Indus, and there, as we learn from his historians, held intercourse with Indian sages. On his death, Persia fell to the share of Seleucus, (307 B.C.) who soon afterwards penetrated even to the Ganges: but being threatened by Antigonus, he entered into an alliance with the Indian Sovereign, Sandracottus (Chundragupta) which was maintained for many years; he even, it is related, gave his daughter in marriage to the Indian sovereign, as well as sent him Grecian auxiliaries to assist in repelling his enemies. Megasthenes and Onesicratus were also sent as an embassy, and the former having resided for some years at Palibothra (Patria), gave the Greeks some of the most correct accounts they had of India. During the reign of the Seleucidæ, and their successors, who held possession of all the countries between the Euphrates, the Indus, and the Oxus, the commerce of India with the North is described as having been very considerable. The recent discovery in the north-western part of ancient India, and in Caubul, of innumerable coins, commencing with the third of the Seleucidæ, and his known successors, and continuing for many centuries, has revealed a series of unrecorded Bactrian princes, who, at first independent, afterwards held sway under the Persian King of Kings over the countries between Persia and India, including some of the north-western provinces of the latter. It is extremely interesting, in this long series of coins, to observe the purely Greek ones succeeded by those having a Greek inscription on one side, and a Pehlevi on the reverse; Native designations, even in Greek characters, becoming substituted for the purely Greek titles; whence the Greek characters are found to have continued in use even until the fourth century, in the provinces of Caubul and the Punjab. From the later Indo-Scythic coins, themselves the continuation of the purely Greek, the Hindoo coinage of Canouge has been clearly proved to have originated by Mr. Prinsep, in his invaluable Journal of the Asiatic Society, vol. 3, 4, and 5. The Parthians, who swayed these Bactrian princes, and who so long and so successfully opposed the Roman arms, made their first attempts 250 B.C. on, and held the Persian sceptre to A.D. 223, when Artaxerxes overthrew their power, and established the Sassanian dynasty, which reigned in Persia from this time to A.D. 632, when the Arabs invaded Persia. During this dynasty, the connexion of Greek physicians with Persia was continued, as some followed the Emperor Valerian, when he was taken prisoner in the year 262 A.D., by Sapor I. Greek physicians were also sent with the daughter of the Emperor Aurelian, when given in marriage to Sapor II., who is said to have built the city of Jondisabour or Nisabur, in honour of his queen. It is related by Dr. Freind, that during the reign of Chosroes, and previous to the embassy from the Romans to Persia of Archindus, who was accompanied by the pseudo-philosopher Uranius, "Damascius the Syrian, Simplicius of Cilicia, Diogenes of Phœnicia, and Isidorus of Gaza, &c., the greatest and most learned philosophers of the age, having an aversion to the established religion, retired into Persia." (1. p. 133). It is thought by some authors, that it was in consequence of the settling of the above Greek physicians at Jondisabour, that this became celebrated as a medical school, and that so many of the more celebrated Arabian physicians, as

Rhazes, Haly Abbas, and Avicenna, were educated in the more eastern parts of Asia.

From this historical review, it is evident that continued communication was maintained between the Greeks and Persians from the time of Ctesias, or the fourth century before, to the sixth century after our Saviour. But this brings the connexion even beyond the time of Oribasius and Ætius, who are noted for having preserved whatever was valuable in what has been called the Egyptian, but which to me looks very like Indian Polypharmacy. These authors having lived in the fourth and fifth centuries, are not much, if at all, anterior to the time of Nooshirwan, when Barzouyeh was sent from Persia into India for medicaments. Previous even to this (A.D. 330), we hear of the Persian king Bahram visiting, in disguise, the Court of Basdeo, sovereign of Canouge, to study the laws, religion, and manners of the Hindoos. To this intercommunication has usually been ascribed the coincidences which have been observed between the science of the Greeks and that of the Hindoos; and it has, therefore, been inferred, that the latter must have borrowed from the former; though the facts, I conceive, are as well calculated to prove the reverse.

As Plants, from their fixedness to the soil, and subjection to the atmosphere, indicate to geologists the climates in which they lived in former ages of the world, even better than animals, which from changes of covering frequently adapt themselves to new situations; so shall we find plants, or such of their products as are applied to medical purposes, well suited to indicate the antiquity of the cultivation of medicine, in the countries where alone we know they can grow. Taking, therefore, the articles of Materia Medica as they were handed to us by the Arabs, we shall find in their names and the countries whence they must ever have been introduced, indications of the different schools of medicine, which have flourished at different times; and all of which find a place in history, except the Indian. Thus the plants and medicines of European climates, of Asia Minor and of Syria, we can account for, from the continued existence of Greek physicians, from the time of Hippocrates to that of Paulus Ægineta; those of Egypt and Africa, from the Alexandrian School, which subsisted from B.C. 300 to A.D. 700, or to the period of the destruction of its institutions by the Arabians. The occurrence of Jewish names may also be accounted for, from many physicians having been of the Jewish nation for a series of ages. The properties of medicinal articles must, in very ancient times, have been investigated in Persia, as their fœtid gum-resins early make their appearance in the records of medicine; and in Dioscorides, we have numerous names of plants as given them by the Magi (προφηται). Jondisabour, also, was a celebrated medical school, previous to the Arabians, as G. Bactishua was educated there, and celebrated as well for his skill in medicine, as for his proficiency in the Persian and Arabian languages; whence he was sent for to attend Almanzor, the second Caliph of the Abbasides, and being detained, translated, at his request, several books of medicine. But even previous to him, an impulse had been given to translations from other languages, as the work called Pandects of Medicine, of Aaron the Presbyter, who lived at Alexandria subsequently to the era of the Hegira, was translated in 683 into Arabic by Masarjawaihas. The Old Testament, moreover, was first translated by Warka, the son of Naefel, who is mentioned in the Koran, and who died in A.D. 612.

Considerable as appears to have been Hindoo medicine, and extensive as no doubt has been the influence of its Materia Medica, the absence of all record of the former in the annals of medicine, can only be accounted for from the geographical position of India with respect to Europe, and the total unacquaintance with the refined language of the former, which prevailed in the latter even to our own day. For when the name of even the most celebrated Hindoo writer presented itself before a modern author writing expressly on the subject, it is passed over without comment or examination—"Scharak Indus, a Rhazeo citatus plane ignotus." (Sprengel. Hist. Rei. Herb. 1. p. 234.) That a Hindoo system of medicine does exist, we know from their numerous books on all branches of that science; that some of these were written prior to the Arabs, we have shewn by their being quoted in the works of the latter. How much earlier than the eighth century the principal of them were composed, we may only hope to ascertain by the progress now making in settling Indian Chronology. But in absence of this it is practicable, as I have stated, to get a conviction of the cultivation of medicine among the Hindoos at still earlier periods, from occasional notices by writers of the West; and we cannot but allow them an early knowledge of the properties of many of the valuable drugs which their country afforded them, when we see the necessarily subsequent employment of the same by the Greeks and Romans.

For this purpose it is not again necessary to notice the Hindoo drugs mentioned in the works of the Arabs, and still less to refer to such of the Greek authors as Actuarius and Myrepsus, who were subsequent to them. But it is advisable to keep in mind, that the Arabs, from their position and communication with the East, must necessarily have had a practical knowledge of the articles imported from India, and described in their works; while the Christian physicians employed as translators in the City of the Caliphs, being equally acquainted with both the Greek and Arabic languages, must have correctly applied the synonymous terms, to such drugs as had been long in use; while those which then began to be first employed, must have been introduced either by new or by their Indian names. In this view the continued chain of authors is very valuable, as each is likely to have been well acquainted with the drugs described by at least his immediate predecessor: Myrepsus, therefore, is useful in forming the connexion with the Arab authors, as well as with Paulus Ægineta, whom they so closely succeeded; while he completes the reference to Ætius and Oribasius.

These authors, however, being chiefly copyists of their predecessors, as well as having for the most part practised as far West as Rome, contain little information which is not found in older works, and few new medicines; though their prescriptions are often almost entirely composed of Indian drugs. Paulus of Ægina, who lived in the seventh century, and was a great traveller, treats particularly, as remarked by Dr. Freind, of the diseases of Women, and in his sixth book gives us, even if we compare him with Celsus, the most perfect account of Surgery, as it stood in the time of the ancients. "The chapter concerning the extraction of Darts and Arrows, &c. contains many excellent rules; and the description he gives of that sort of weapon, then in use among the ancients, particularly the Egyptians, is very curious, and clear, as well as concise." (1. p. 163). He notices few new medicines, but, among the Plasters, there is an "Emplastrum indicum;"—"he is probably the first to mention the internal use of Steel, as he speaks much of its virtues in scirrhus of the spleen, and recommends it both in infusion and in substance;" he seems also to have been the first to take notice of Cloves, and of Rhubarb, by the name of "rheum barbaricum," which Actuarius, and after him Myrepsus, called "*reon indicon*,"

Fr. I. p. 82-115. He has also a "Collyrium mitigatorium Trypherum," (p. 169); and a "Smegma aut pulvis egregius: vocant autem quidam ipsum Indum, alii Asclepium;" and of which the prescription is given, as "Descriptio pulveris Indici;" respecting which he observes, "Hic pulvis præstantissimus est et efficax." (Med. artis princip. p. 305. ed. Steph.)

Ætius, a native of Amida, in Mesopotamia, who lived at the end of the fifth century, and studied at Alexandria, must, from his connexions, have had means for obtaining more correct information on eastern subjects. He is most full and original on surgical subjects; much so on both the actual and potential cautery, describing the several ways of making the latter, as well as issues. "He employs nearly a whole book upon plasters, including all those known to the Persians, Egyptians, and Greeks;" and appears to have had some acquaintance with the medicines, diseases, and practice of the East, as he has a "Collyrium Indiarum," mentions Sandaracha (Sulphuret of Arsenic) by its Persian name *Zarnach*; states that "Presbyteri Indi" prepare "pharmacum ad calculos, quod itidem externum lapidem in grumos resolvere posse quidam aiunt." *Nuces Indicæ*, Cocoa-nuts, *Zador*,* (*Zudwar*) and *Galanga* (Sansc. *Kolinjana*), Zedoary and Galangal roots, *Santalum*, Sandalwood, all Indian tropical products are mentioned, for the first time; as well as the fruit of *Semecarpus Anacar-*

* As this prescription is as well calculated as any to give a notice of their nature, and the number of Indian articles usually introduced, it is here transcribed—"Zador id est zedoariæ, galangæ, ligustici, seselis, cardamomi, piperis longi, piperis albi, cinnamomi, zingiberis, seminis Smyrnii, caryophylli, phylli, stachyos, myrobalani, phu, costi, scordii, silphii sive laserpitii, rhei barbarici, pæoniæ, alii etiam arboris nucis viscum et paliuri semen, itemque saxifragum ac casiam addunt; ex his singulis stateres duos commisceto. Datur cum condito aut vino vetere ad balneum ituris, et sine balneo vespere, similiterque mane." In the "Suffumigii moschati præparatio," there are also numerous, if not all Indian products.

dium, in the "Antidotus Theodoretos ex Anacardiis;" though the introduction of these, as well as of musk and of ambergris, is usually referred to the Arabs. It is remarkable, that he states, "Qui nunc ab omnibus Lobi nominantur apud omnes veteres dolichi et phaseoli appellantur." In India, at the present day, one of the most common of the pulses, a species of *Dolichos*, is called *lobia*, which, in all dictionaries, is marked as a Persian word. There is also an "Antidotus ex duobus piperis generibus," from Archigenes, who seems also to have had considerable knowledge of the East. He was a Syrian, practised at Rome, wrote much on medicine, and is alluded to by Juvenal more than once. A well-known Indian disease, "Elephantiasis a quibusdam leontiasis, ab aliis satyriasis appellatur," is described in Ætius from Archigenes. "Regio vero hujus mali inductrix est tum quæ valde calida est, tum quæ vehementer frigida." Among the remedies, we have "Eboris etiam et cornu cervini ramenta;" and we have it stated that "In regione Indorum elephantiasi affectos, assidue per sedem eluere per urinæ asininæ infusionem heminæ mensura calefactæ consueverunt. Crocodilium item terrestrem accipiunt, et magnum sane testimonium de hoc remedio præbent." Among the remedies we have also "Myrobalanus item cum aceto præstat: probe auxiliatur et alumen cum sale et sandaracha æquis partibus in vino et oleo, maxime lentiscino, aut si non adsit, rosaceo tritis." Ætius quotes Leonides, for another complaint common in India, that is, the Dracunculi, or guinea-worms, which he says, "Nascuntur autem hi in Æthiopia ac India."

Oribasius, though born at Pergamus, is usually styled a Sardian, from having studied probably at Sardes, in the school of Zeno the Cyprian, who afterwards removed to Alexandria. He was not only the countryman, but also the copyist, of Galen, of whose Materia Medica, as well as of that of Dioscorides, he has given an alphabetical epitome, arranged under the heads of plants, minerals, and animals. Among these I do not perceive any articles not known to his predecessors. Galen himself, though so voluminous a writer, takes his Materia Medica almost entirely from Dioscorides; and though sufficiently interested in the subject to have visited Cœlo-Syria to see the Balsam-tree, I find no drugs which are not contained in the work of the former. Indian medicines are, however, abundantly prescribed in the compounds which he enumerates, and among them, some which are called Indian, as "Indicum Tharsei chirurgi emplastrum.—Ceræ, resinæ frictæ, picis aridæ, bituminis liquidi Zacynthii, singulorum lib. ij. cerussæ, æruginis, chalictedis, misyos peregrini, melanteriæ, aluminis et scissilis et rotundi, gallæ omphacitidis, malicorii, rhei, thuris, singulorum silibram, aceti quantum sufficit;" also, "Collyrium Indicum ærianum inscriptum;" and "Indicum basilicon inscriptum indicus lapis:"—that Indian medicines were much used in Rome, even prior to his time, we know from Pliny, who inveighs against their introduction: "Arabia atque India in medio æstimantur, ulcerique parvo medicina a Rubro Mare imputatur."

From Pliny we might adduce numerous instances of the knowledge which the ancients possessed of the natural productions of India, but as his information is chiefly derived from earlier sources, it will be better introduced when we have to notice these. But in his account of the country and climate, the names of towns and rivers, as well as in his description of the animals and plants of India, we find much correct information intermixed with monstrous fables. This naturally diminishes our faith in the other parts of his statement: but as a natural historian, he seems to have thought it necessary to repeat what he found related, even when he shews that he does not himself believe the statements. In his accounts of the plants and articles of Materia Medica, he chiefly follows Theophrastus and Dioscorides; those not described by them are almost entirely European plants. It is interesting, for our purpose of investigating the origin and connexions of ancient medicine, to find him mentioning many Egyptian medicines, and giving the opinions respecting others of the Persian Magi. The art of magic, he says, "Natam primum e medicina nemo dubitat;" and "pariter utrasque artes effloruisse medicinam dico, magicenque, eadem ætate illam Hippocrate hanc Democrito illustrantibus, circa Peloponnesiacum Græciæ bellum:" lib. 30. c. 1. and 3. In proceeding to the description and uses of precious stones, he further says, "Nunc gemmarum confessa genera dicemus, a laudatissimis orsi. Nec vero id solum agemus, sed ad majorem utilitatem vitæ obiter coarguetur Magorum infanda vanitas, quando illi vel plurima prodidere de gemmis, medicinæ ex his blanda specie prodigia transgressi." 37. c. xiv. Gems and precious stones we have seen (p. 4. and 54) were also employed by the Hindoos as medicines; many of those dilated on even by Persians, must then, as now, have been procured from India. This must also have been the case with those described by Pliny; as indeed he has mentioned in numerous places, besides saying, "Gemmiferæ amnes sunt Acesines et Ganges; terrarum autem omnium maxime India." lib. 37. c. 76.

Galen and Pliny having both borrowed much from Dioscorides, the most celebrated, as well as the most copious author on the Materia Medica of the Ancients, it is necessary for our purpose to consider more fully the parts of his work having reference to India, since, from his eastern connexions, he was able to procure more full and more correct information, especially after the increased trade which took place with India by the Red Sea, subsequent to the foundation of Alexandria. "The numerous copper coins of Egyptian fabrication, found in India, confirms what is known from history of that country having been the principal channel of commerce between India and the Roman empire." (J. A. S.) To these causes must be chiefly ascribed the information we find in Dioscorides, who was a native of Anazarbus, in Cilicia, and probably studied at Tarsus, the capital of that province, as well as visited Alexandria and the North of Africa, and also Spain, France, and Italy. He must have lived in the early part of the first century, as in his preface he mentions Licinius Bassus, who was consul in A.D. 63. He was probably contemporary with, as he is so frequently quoted, though never named by Pliny; but appears to be alluded to in the passage, where, after transcribing the account of Schistus by the former, Pliny adds, "hanc esse sententiam eorum qui nuperrime scripserint."

Dioscorides is, besides, the most ancient author who has written expressly, at the same time that he has done so most fully, on Materia Medica, a subject to which he was so much attached, as to have travelled in many countries, and to have followed the Roman armies for its investigation. His work, therefore, is the best calculated to shew how much the ancients were indebted to India and the East for their medicines; especially as he assists us in identifying them by introducing some degree of arrangement, as well as by describing their physical properties with their medical uses. He is particular also in giving many synonymes, as well as in specifying the countries where they were severally produced. Taking, therefore, those which are stated to be of Indian origin, we are struck by finding some of them also mentioned as being the produce of Syria and Media; but this is easily explained by our knowing that the products of the East reached the West both by the Red

Sea, Arabia, and Egypt, as by the Euphrates, and through the desert-surrounded Palmyra to Syria. Hence the last place of export, as is the case even in the present day, came to be considered as the country actually producing the drug.

The majority of Indian articles are arranged by Dioscorides in his first book, among aromatics, for which India has always been, and still is famed. Among these are the substances already mentioned at p. 33, as *Nardos*, which is no doubt *Nardostachys* (*Patrinia*, Don) *Jatamansi*, D.C., which I have procured from the very mountains, where it is described by Dioscorides as growing—" Quæ Gangitis appellatur, a fluvio quodam, cui Ganges nomen, montem prætercurrente in quo nascitur." The Syrian and Mountain kinds, the latter called also *sampharetica*, are thought by Sprengel in Diosc. ed. Kuhn II. p. 346, to be, the first—*Patrinia scabiosæfolia* Fisch., found in Dahuria; and the second—*Valeriana Hardwickii*. The roots of the latter are still used in medicine in Nepal and N. India, being imported into the latter from the Himalayan mountains. Σχοινος (sometimes written Σχινος, but which is the mastic-tree) very distinct from the Σχοινος ελεια of the fourth book, c. 52, is usually translated *Juncus odoratus*, and is universally allowed to be *Andropogon Schœnanthus*, or Lemon-grass. *Calamus Aromaticus* (v. p. 33) is, I conceive, *Andropogon Calamus Aromaticus*, nob., which covers the extensive arid plains of Central India, a country interspersed with large and numerous lakes, and therefore resembling that described by Theophrastus, as the country where this " sweet Calamus" grows. Some authors, as Sprengel, &c., suppose that this is the plant now called *wuj* in Arabic, the *Acorus Calamus* of botanists; but of this Arabian authors give *akoron*, as the Greek name, and apply to it the description by Dioscorides of ακορος, which this plant no doubt is. *Wuj* is itself derived from the Sanscrit *vacha*, as is the common Hindee name, *buch*, by which, in Indian bazars, I obtained the roots of *Acorus Calamus;* one of the *Aroideæ*, and very different from the most fragrant of grasses, as is that of Namur.

The other species of καλαμος, Diosc. 1. 114, is translated *arundo*, and by the Arabs *kusb*, under which they arrange the different kinds of bamboo, which were probably included under the general denomination by Dioscorides. This we may infer, from solid or male and female kinds being mentioned, as well as their uses for pipes, arrows, and for writing; for which these, with species of *Arundo* and *Saccharum*, are now employed in India. Allied to these in a botanical point of view, is *Saccharum officinarum*, which has needlessly been supposed not to have yielded *saccharum*, or the substance known by this name to the ancients; the same authors conjecturing this to be *Tabasheer*, now so well known as found within the bamboo. Considering that this substance is pure *silex*, it is not likely to have been arranged with the honeys, and described under the head of περι Σακχαρου μελιτος. The Arabic name, moreover, of sugar, is *sukkur*, derived from the Sanscrit *sarkura*, or Tamul *sakkara*.

Under κυπειρος, *Cyperus rotundus*, L., a second kind is described as the produce of India (*Cyperus indicus*, Auct.). The Arabs give *sād* as the synonyme of *Cyperus*; and, in India, *motha*, Sans. *moostha*, is given as the synonyme of *sād;* and we obtain, under that name, the roots of *Cyperus hexastychus*, Rottb., a species which, was considered by Dr. Roxburgh to be identical with *C. rotundus*. The irregular-formed tubers, about the size of acorns, which constitute the root, are eaten by cattle in India, and used as a perfume at the weddings of the natives.

In noticing the various productions of India, supposed to have been known to the ancients, it is interesting to observe how many of these are the produce of the Peninsula, and of the neighbouring island of Ceylon; for it is to these parts historians have shewn that the earliest trade was directed from Arabia, Egypt, and the Red Sea. Among the principal of these products is Cinnamon, *κινναμωμον*, often written *κιναμον*, corrupted into *akimona*, in Persian works, of which the Cingalese *cacyn-nama*, (*dulce lignum*), or the Malayan *kaimanis*, appear to have been the original; as Herodotus says, "quos nos petentes a Phœnicibus cinnamomon vocamus." The Arabic name is *dar-seeni*, evidently derived from the Hindee *dar-chinee*, of which *daroosita* is said to be the Sanscrit. Cinnamon is produced by *Cinnamomum zeylanicum*. But if we infer from the name, that the Hindoos first became acquainted with Cinnamon from China, *C. aromaticum* of Cochin-China and the southern provinces of that country, yields a Cinnamon, by some considered nearly equal to that of Ceylon. The Cassia of the ancients it is not easy to determine: that of commerce, Mr. Marshall says consists of only the inferior kinds of Cinnamon. Some consider Cassia to be distinguished from Cinnamon, by the outer cellular covering of the bark being scraped off the latter, but allowed to remain on the former. (Thomson Dispen.) This is, however, the characteristic of the bark of the above-named *C. aromaticum*; as we are informed by Mr. Crawford, that it is not cured like that of Ceylon, by freeing it from the epidermis (Emb. to Siam. p. 470). —The Arabians consider Cassia to be their *sulikhe*, probably the *selackal* or *'sindoc* bark of Amboyna, produced by *Cinnamomum Culitlawan*, or by *C. Sintoc* of Blume, if this be distinct from the former. *C. nitidum*, the *koolit-manis* of Sumatra, has bark with the taste and smell of Cinnamon. Some species are peculiar to the Peninsula of India; and one, Dr. Hamilton informs us, yields a kind of Cassia in Canara. Considering that besides these, there are other species of this genus with aromatic bark, and that ten varieties are described of both the Ceylon and China Cinnamon, it will not appear surprising that we are unable to distinguish accurately the *Canella, Cassia lignea*, and *Cassia fistula*, or *achy, sigir, mosylites, aphysemon, kitto, dacar*, as the varieties of Cassia, nor *mosylon, xylocinnamomum, xylodes*, &c. as those of Cinnamon. It is not an accidental coincidence, that both ancients and moderns mention a great variety of each; but none as growing elsewhere than in southern latitudes. Another produce of the same family is the *Malabathrum* leaf of the ancients (v. p. 82), which appears to be a corrupted form of writing *Tamala-patra* (Tamala leaf.) This, in Arabic works, is described under the name *saduj*, with *malatroon* as the Greek, and *tuj* and *tej-pat* as the Hindee synonymes. By the latter names may be obtained every where in the bazars of India, the leaves of *Cinnamomum Tamala* and of *C. albiflorum*; being as commonly used there as *bay-leaves* are in Europe. Their being brought out of the forests stript from the branches, or picked up after they have fallen, may have given origin to the fables with which their early accounts were accompanied.

These leaves having frequently been described simply as *Folium* or *Folium indicum*; some authors have been led (v. Bodæus in Theophr. p. 1035) to suppose, that they might be the *betel*-leaf or *pan* of the Hindoos, Pers. *tumbol*, Ar. *tunbol*, Sans. *tumbolee*, the produce of *Piper Betle*, which is extensively cultivated in all the southern parts of India. The plant has probably been introduced from some of the Tropical Islands (*India aquosa* of old writers), as no botanist has yet found it in a wild state in Continental India. Being used by the natives in its fresh state, it is not likely to have been an article of commerce to the West. So, *Cubebs*, *kubabeh* of the Arabs, and *kubab-chini* of the

Hindoos, produced by *Piper Cubeba*, also a native of the Indian Archipelago, has been thought to be the *Carpesium* of the Greeks, because it was so of the Arabs; but the description does not apply, and the geographical distribution of the plant is beyond the range of those which seem alone to have been known to the Greeks. The knowledge of the others may have been introduced into India in an age subsequent to that when the Greeks were best acquainted with that country. This is probable, from their having been so well accodinted with the indigenous species of Pepper; as *Piper nigrum* must then, as now, have yielded both black and white pepper, as *P. longum* does long pepper. The root of the latter also, so extensively used in India as a stimulant medicine, and called *pippula-mool*, is, no doubt, the πεπεριως ριζα, though Sprengel says, "Quid radicem piperis veteres vocarint, non liquet." The Sanscrit *pippulee*, (Hindee *pippul*, Pers. *pilpil*, Ar. *filfil*,) is, no doubt, the origin of the Greek πεπερι. In all the above languages, the adiuncts, black or round, white and long, are added, to distinguish the different kinds; but the natives of India alone have distinct names, *mirch*, (Sansc. *mircha*), for *P. nigrum*, and *pippul* for *P. longum*.

After the Peppers, and described by Pliny as "*sapore simile*," is mentioned an equally well-known Indian plant; this is Ζιγγιβερις, or *Zingiber*, of which the name, like the Arab. *Zinjabil*, Pers. *Shungveer*, is derived from the Sansc. *Shringuverum*, as has been shewn by Mr. Colebrooke. *Zingiber officinale*, the plant, is cultivated in the plains of Bengal, as well as at elevations of from 3,000 to 4,000 feet in 30° N. latitude. As its crop depends upon the root, which is pro tated by the earth from great vicissitudes of temperature, this may, with irrigation, be cultivated further north than is practicable with other tropical plants; and it is described as having been so in Egypt. In the same family with the Ginger, is the Cardamom plant, *Elettaria* or *Alpinia Cardamomum*, found only in the mountains of the Malabar coast. It has been doubted whether our Cardamoms are those which were known to the ancients, and of which several kinds are mentioned by Pliny by this name. They have been considered such from the time of the Arabs, who describe them under the names of *kakleh* and *khyrboa*, and distinguish the large from the small kind. They also keep distinct their translation of *kirdamana*, the *cardaminen* or *Sisymbrium alterum* of Dioscorides, which has been confounded with Cardamoms by some of the older commentators.

There is a produce of this family which one is surprised was not known to the Greeks. This is Turmeric, or the tubers of *Curcuma longa*, so universally employed, and apparently from the highest antiquity, both as a medicine and as a condiment, in every part of India. The Latin name is evidently derived from *kurkum*, the Persian name for saffron, Ar. *zafran*. Some authors, indeed, suppose that the ancient saffron was turmeric. This, by the Arabs, is called *arook-al-safr*, or yellow root. The French formerly called it *Terra-merita* (Curcuma, hæc Gallis Terra merita male dicitur), and the Portuguese *Soffran da Terra*, as well as *Crocus indicus*. Some have supposed Turmeric to be the *Cyperus indicus* of Dioscorides, and his description in some measure warrants the inference, as Pliny, apparently copying the passage, says, "Est et per se Indica herba, quæ cyperis vocatur, zingiberis effigie: commanducata croci vino reddit." From the colour and form, this root would appear to have been known to the ancients, as, indeed, must have been inferred by the Arabians, who give, as its Greek synonyme, *khaldoonion tomagha*, evidently a corruption of χελιδόνιον το μεγα, but the colour of the juice alone agrees with the description of the plant by Dioscorides.

Costus, of which three kinds are described, Arabian, Syrian, and Indian, the produce of these several countries; is called *kust* by the Arabs, with *koostus* assigned as the Greek, *koshta* as Syriac, and *kooth* as the Hindee name. By the latter I obtained two kinds in the bazars of N. India, one called *koost-tulkh* and *koost-hindee*, Indian or bitter *Costus*, and the other *koost-sheeren*, also *koost-buhree* and *Arabee*, that is, Arabian or sweet *Costus*, this having a fragrant odour, resembling that of iris root; but I was unable to trace out either the country or the plant which produced it, though it was said to be brought into India from Caubul and Cashmere. On comparing this sweet Costus with the specimens of Materia Medica I collected in Calcutta, I cannot distinguish it from a root well known in the market there by the name of *Puchuk*. This identity was long ago ascertained by Garcias ab Horto, as he says, "Est ergo Costus dictus Arabibus *Cost* aut *Cast*: in Guzerate Vplot, in Malaca ubi ejus plurimus est usus, *Pucho*, et inde vehitur in Sinarum regionem."—"Nascitur circa Guzarate, inter Bengalea, Delli, et Cambaya, in Mandou et Chitor." Clus. Exot. lib. 1. c. 35. On referring to Macculloch's Com. Dict. and Milburn's Orient. Com., I find *Putchook* described as the "root of a plant growing in Sinde, and imported in considerable quantities from the north-west coast of India into China. When burned it yields a fine smell. The Chinese beat it into a fine powder, which they burn as incense in the temples of their gods."

Another product of India known to the ancients, and still employed by the Chinese as an incense, is *Agallochum*, Lign-aloe, or eagle-wood, *pao-d'agila*, and *pao-d'aquila* of the Portuguese, names, no doubt, derived from the Malayan *agila*, which in Sanscrit is *agura*, Hindee *aggur*, but which the Arabs know by the name *aod hindee.* Of this, there are two kinds; the Indian is the produce of *Aquilaria Agallocha*, Roxb. (Royle Illustr. Him. Bot. Tab. 36. f. 1.) abundant in the forests of Silhet and Chittagong, and probably extending into the Burmese territories. *Calambac*, or the Cochin-Chinese kind of *Agallochum*, is that produced by *Aloexylum Agallochum* of Loureiro. Nothing can be more inapplicable to the descriptions of Lign-aloe, than any part of the genus Aloe, which is often referred to as yielding this fragrant wood. The mistake Sprengel supposes may have arisen from one of the Arabic names, *allowat* or *allieh*, having been converted into *αλοην*. Aloes is probably derived from *elwa*, the common Hindee name for aloes (Ar. *sibbur*), which is produced by *Aloe vulgaris*, and other species, in Africa, India, and Arabia. It would be easier to contend, as has sometimes been done, that the Lign-aloe of the ancients is the Sandal-wood of India (Pers. *sundul*, Hind. *chundun*, Sans. *chandana*, Tamul, *shandana*). The tree *Santalum album* is a native of the Malabar coast, where the best is produced; and it is possible, from the fragrant nature of the wood, that it may have been thought a kind of *Agallochum*, or Lign-aloe; but Arab authors keep distinct its description.

Ebony is a product of the Malabar coast, which has been known from the earliest times, and its name appears of eastern origin, as, in India it is called *abnoos*. It was also, and no doubt still is, produced in Abyssinia, though we have no recent botanical testimony on the subject; but both Maillet and Burkhardt mention it as one of the articles brought by the caravans into Egypt. *Diospyros Ebenus* yields the best kind in the Mauritius, perhaps, also, in Madagascar: but *D. Ebenaster* and *D. melanoxylon*, the ebony-trees of the Coromandel coast, yield it in the Peninsula, of very good quality, as other species do in other parts of India.

Bdellium is another Indian product described by Dioscorides, who gives *madelcon* and *bolchon* as other names. This the Persian authors describe under *mokl*, giving *budleeon* and *madikon* as its Greek, and *googul* as its Hindee synonymes, stating it to be produced by the Doom Palm (*Cucifera thebaica*). The *googul* obtained in N. India I was told was the product of a tree, which, from its birch-like bark and other characters, I knew to be the *Amyris* (now *Balsamodendron*) *Agallocha* of Dr. Roxburgh; which he, almost at the other extremity of India, had also been informed was called *googula*. This he describes to be a native of the districts of Silhet and Assam, diffusing, when bruised, a grateful fragrance, like that of the finest myrrh. This *googul* must be a very different substance from the *gogul* described as a species of Bitumen, used at Bombay, Bengal, &c., for painting the bottoms of ships (Milb. Or. Com. p. 102). The African *Bdellium*, probably the *mokl-al-mukkee*, *Bdellium mechium* of Avicenna, is produced by *Heudelotia africana* (Arch. de Bot. 1. p. 421), another of the *Terebinthaceæ;* Avicenna describes one of the kinds, as *mokl-al-yahoodee*, or *Bdellium judaicum*.

Olibanum, from λιβανος (Arab. *looban*), the *thus* of the ancients, is another fragrant resin, of which both an Arabian and an Indian variety are described: two kinds continue to be known in modern as in ancient commerce. The tree producing the first kind has not yet been ascertained, but it may be a native both of Africa and Arabia (v. Spr. in Diosc. 11. p. 376). The Indian kind, which is called *koondur*, and under which name *Olibanum* is described by the Arabs, has been shewn by Mr. Colebrooke to be the produce of *Boswellia serrata* v. *thurifera*. I have taken some off the tree, which closely, though not exactly, resembles that of commerce, burning with a highly grateful perfume. The only other Indian product certainly made out is *Lycium indicum*, v. p. 32. Garcias supposed this to be the *Cate* or *Catechu* of the present day, but there is no proof of its having been such. It is, however, remarkable, that *Catechu* is not noticed among the substances known to the ancients; but it may have been confounded with some other astringent, as *Acacia;* or having so long been called *Terra Japonica*, it may be elsewhere described; as Indigo is among mineral substances. (Diosc. v. c. 107.)

Two substances alone of those stated to be Indian products, have not yet been ascertained. Of these, *Narcaphthon*, or *Nascaphthon*, has been supposed to be Mace; as *Cancamum*, described as the exudation of an Arabian tree, has been conjectured to be the lac (*lūk*) dye and resin of India. *Macer*, a bark from the Barbaric region, has been thought to be *Wrightia antidysenterica*, supposing this to be the *macre*, described by Crist. d'Acosta, of the Brahmans on the Malabar coast, (Clus. Exot. p. 266). Though *Macer* is always described as a bark, I had given me as such the highly aromatic leaves of *Rhododendron lepidotum*, under the name of *talisfur*. *Mafur* and *mafurboos* (the *f.* is easily changed into *k.* v. p. 32) are, in Persian works, assigned as the Greek names of *talisafar*, under which name, the *Macer* of Dioscorides is alluded to by Avicenna. *Amomum* is another substance, which still remains unknown, but for which the Asiatics give a substitute, if it be not the original substance. It is remarkable, that under the name *humama*, I obtained the same plant, composed entirely of a cluster of small leaves, which Clusius has figured Exot. lib. 1. c. 31. p. 199. as *humama* sent him from Ormuz; and which Sprengel has supposed to be *Forstera magellanica*, brought by Sir F. Drake.

From the foregoing enumeration, in which I have confined myself to those substances expressly mentioned as being procured from India, we perceive how largely the Greeks were indebted to that country for their Materia Medica. From the tropical latitudes and climates in which alone these substances can flourish, we may infer the early populousness and civilisation of these countries, as well as the extent to which ancient commerce reached, independent of historical testimony on the subject. That the Greeks were still more indebted to eastern nations, might also be shewn by numerous articles, which are, and from the dependence of vegetation on climate, must ever have been the produce of the East. Of many of these the original oriental names have, with slight alterations, passed into the Greek, and been the source also of the European names of these substances.

Without dwelling on the early employment of *Galbanum*, *Assafœtida*, *Ammoniacum*, *Sagapenum*, and *Opoponax*, the products of Persia, and therefore, indicating the antiquity of their investigation in that country, as well as of the nations by whom their use was adopted, there are others of which the names prove their oriental origin;—as *kumoon*, *Cuminum*; *kinnub*, *Cannabis*; *kibbur*, *Capparis*; *koorkum*, *Crocus*; *koortum*, *Carthamus*; *semsem*, *Sesamum*; *yasmin*, *Jasminum*; *sosun*, *Susinum*, Diosc. 1. c. 62; *nurgus*, *Narcissus*; *hoormul*, *Harmala*; *molee*, *Moly*; *belessan*, *Balsamum*; *moor*, *Myrrha*; *mun*, *Manna*; *sukmoonia*, *Scammonia*; *pista*, *Pistacia*; *kurseea*, *κερασος*, *Cerasus*; *burkook*, *Præcocia*; the last is also called *mala armeniaca*; but this, and the names of some of the other fruits, as *mala medica* and *persica*, point out at once the countries whence they became known to the ancients.

Besides these, there are many others, which we know were early employed as medicinal agents, as the Pomegranate (Arabic *rōman*, Greek *ροας*), of which the bark of the root, the rind of the fruit, and both the single and double flowers are employed in oriental, as in Greek medicine. I do not know whether it be an accidental circumstance, that the purgative root of *Pityusa* has *turpet* assigned as a synonyme, as this is remarkable for its resemblance to *turbud*, the root of *Convolvulus Turpethum*. Many also of the *Cucurbitaceæ*, *Umbelliferæ*, and *Labiatæ*, are common to the Materia Medica of the East, as well as to that of the West; but to dwell further on these is unnecessary.

In examining the list of articles enumerated, as imported by the Greeks from India, there are some substances now extremely common and extensively used there, which one would expect to find among those first known to strangers, as Turmeric and Catechu, already mentioned; so also, Turbith, Galangal, Zedoary, and Zerumbet, as well as Sandal-wood and Areca-nut. Some of these may have been known by other names, or confounded with other substances. Such poisons as *bish*, *Aconitum ferox*, and *Strychnos Nux vomica*, the ancients seem to have been unacquainted with; but some trace of them may be found when the works of the Hindoos on poisons and their antidotes, are compared with the oldest works on such subjects in the literature of the West, as that of the Poet Nicander; for both Egypt and India were celebrated for their poisons, as early even as the time of Theophrastus (lib. ix. c. 15).

If it excite surprise that some of these were unknown to the ancients, there are others, of which the absence is significant of the extent to which commerce and navigation had advanced, at the times when the other articles were well known; as, for instance, Camphor, Cloves, Nutmeg, Mace, Benzoin, Betel-leaf, Cubebs, Croton Tiglium, Gamboge, &c., all of which are so remarkable in nature, that we could hardly fail in recognising them, if they were described at all like those which have been enumerated as the produce of India or its islands. The others, being produced only in more southern tropical islands, were probably in those days but imperfectly, if at all known in India: or the supply might not, in addition to their own demands, be sufficient for export; or this might not be desirable, when they had so many indigenous products, suited to the wants of those who visited or traded with the Peninsula of India.

The animals mentioned by Dioscorides not being exclusively confined to India, do not afford the same kind of argument that we have derived from plants; especially as the want of precision in the identity of the species described, and those existing in India, as well as the extent of distribution of the latter have not yet been ascertained; yet we may obtain some corroboration of the inferences deduced from plants. Thus, though the African Elephant may have yielded its spoils to form the ivory of the ancients, Peacocks could have been procured from India only. The Cantharides, described by Dioscorides, are species of *Mylabris*, and *M. Cichorei* is that now most commonly employed in India. The *Scincus*, stated to be a native of both Egypt and India, is considered to be *Scincus officinalis*; a similar species is employed in medicine in the north of India in the present day. From the descriptions of Εχιδνης, *viperæ*, it may be inferred that some of those of southern latitudes were known to the ancients. The Asiatic kind, mentioned by Nicander and Galen, is supposed to be *Coluber ægyptius* (Spreng.) *Castor*, the *joondbeduster* of the Arabs, being called *καστορος* by the Greeks, it is curious to find the name *kustooree* applied to the musk animal in the Himalayas, where this is abundant, and constantly hunted for its valuable musk-bag. Ονυξ, usually translated *Unguis odoratus*, and *Blatta Bizantia*, (the operculum of *Strombus lentiginosus*, but which is less fragrant than that of *Pleurotoma Babyloniæ* or *Pl. Trapezii*), is described as being brought from the *nard-producing lakes*. This may every where be obtained in Northern India by the Arabic name *azfar-al-teeb*, though I was unable to ascertain whence it was brought. I am informed by Professor Wilson, that *nakhi*, literally *nail*, is enumerated amongst perfumes in the *Amera Cosha*, and that it is common in the bazars, and procurable by that name in Bengal. Pearls are well known to have been procured in ancient times, as now, from the Persian Gulf and the western coast of Ceylon. Corals, sponges, and cuttle-fish bone, may be found in the bazars of India, as articles of Materia Medica; as well as *lapis judaicus* (*hijr-al-yahoodee*) the calcareous olive-shaped spine of a fossil Echinus. Among these we should expect to find some notice of the Lac insect, and its valuable dye and useful resin. It was certainly known to the Arabian authors by the name لوك, *lūk* or *luch*. By the translators of Avicenna, it was considered identical with the *Cancamum* of Dioscorides: but if so, it is remarkable that, acquainted as the Arabians were with Chermes (from *kirm*, a worm), no mention should be made of the remarkable colouring property of this substance, difficult though this may be of extraction. Dr. Bancroft states, it "was probably unknown in Europe, until after the Portuguese had visited India, by sailing round the Cape of Good Hope." Phil. of Perm. Colours. v. ii. p. 1.

If we adopt with minerals the same method as with vegetables and animals, that is, shew from their being the products of the country, that they were likely to have been known to its inhabitants, and to be identical with the substances described in their works, however ancient these may be: it is necessary to premise, that we cannot always draw the same inferences from their being used in other latitudes, as we may do with substances produced by the organic kingdom, because their distribution is uninfluenced by climate. It is well known that under the equator, as in polar regions, we may have rocks identical in composition, as in their mineral and metallic treasures. But still some inferences may be deduced even from them, and it is incumbent, in contending for the original investigation of the properties of such substances, to shew, at least, that the Hindoos had the means within themselves, or by communication with their immediate neighbours, of becoming acquainted with such substances, independent of the civilisation, or even existence, of distant nations.

Owing to the peculiarity of the soil in many places, and the dryness of the climate in some parts of the year, many of the salts known as mineral substances in other parts of the world, are found in India effloresced in considerable quantities on the surface, or may be washed out of the soil with comparatively little labour or expense. Most have been already mentioned, as saltpetre and nitrate of lime, carbonate of soda, sulphate of soda, and also of magnesia; so also common salt on the banks of the Jumna, and on the shores of the Samur lake. Though sal-ammoniac and alum are manufactured, and the latter even imported from China, native sulphate of alumine is found in considerable quantities in Nepal, as also in Behar; and sal-ammoniac in Persia, near Basman, where it is called *koh-nuoshadur*, as well as in Chinese Tartary and Khoten (J.A.S. iv. p. 659.) Carbonate of magnesia has been found in considerable quantities in the Peninsula, though it has probably never been used medicinally. Carbonate of lime is common every where, either in the form of the calcareous concretion called *kunkur*, or as limestone, both in the mountains of the Peninsula and in those of the Himalayas. In the latter, it is associated both with gypsum and with sulphate of barytes in the neighbourhood of Mussooree. *Tincana*, the Sanscrit name for borax, is no doubt the origin of the Persian *tinkar*, and of the English tincal. An artificial compound, extensively used in India as a medicine, may be mentioned with the above substances: this is the salt commonly called *bit-noben* or *bit-loben*, and black salt (*kala nimuk*), which consists of muriate of soda, oxide of iron, and some impurities. There is some difficulty in ascertaining the identity of all the above substances, with those known to Dioscorides; but it is interesting to remark, that all those which are now produced in Egypt, are also so in India. The ancients were no doubt acquainted with argol and potash, impure Bitartrate and Carbonate of Potass., as τρυξ seu Fæx vini, Diosc. v. c. 13. must have afforded the former, and τεφρα κληματινης, or Sarmentorum cinis, Diosc. v. c. 134, the latter. The *Sal indus* of old authors, has, by some commentators, been thought to be sugar, and by others to be *Tabasheer*; but it has not yet been definitively determined.

Many earthy minerals were employed by the Greeks, and are described in the works of the Arabs; none are, however, stated to be the produce of India; most, indeed, were obtained in the Mediterranean region. Some are found in Indian bazars, no doubt introduced in consequence of the prevalent use of Persian translations of Arab Medical works; but the different ochres and clays do not afford distinctive enough characters to enable us always to recognise them by the short descriptions appended to their names. The substance in the present day known as Red Earth, or Indian Red, is obtained from the islands of the Persian Gulf. *Talc*, introduced by this name into medicine by the Arabians, is supposed to be the *Terra Samia* of the ancients; *Mica*, in plates, is given as *Talc* in India; it is mentioned in the oldest Hindoo works by the name *abruk*, and is found in abundance in Central India.

Of combustible minerals, the Diamond, procured from the mines of Panna and of Golconda, may be considered as almost peculiar to India. Sulphur, found in Cutch, in the Peninsula, and in Nepal, is imported also from the East-India islands, as well as from those of the Persian Gulf. Plumbago is found both in Ceylon and the Himalayas. Ambery (which the Arabs call *kahroba*, grass attractor) is dug up in Cutch, and in the Hukong valley on the S.E. of Assam. Ambergrise is found on the eastern seas and the coast of Madagascar. The Sanscrit *Ambara* is no doubt the origin of both terms, though the first was early known in Europe by other names. Asphaltum is found near the Dead Sea: it is called by the Arabs *kufr-al-yayoodee*, the translation of *bitumen judaicum*. Jet is procured both in Ceylon and China. Of mineral oils, naphtha is found in large quantities, both in Persia and near Rangoon, in Burma. Petroleum is said to be found in Silhet.

Of metallic minerals, the abundance is great in different parts of India, and must always have afforded the Hindoos the means of procuring the several metals in a pure state. Gold has been long washed out of sand, both in the Peninsula of India and along the foot of the Himalaya. Silver occurs in the Malayan Peninsula, but the great portion of both in India must have consisted of the tribute paid by all nations, as well for its natural riches as manufacturing skill. The ores of iron, copper, and lead, are abundant, both in Southern and Central India; also in the Himalayan mountains. Indian *Wootz* has long been celebrated, and Mr. Wilkinson has ingeniously shewn that the figuring of the genuine Damascus blades depends upon the peculiar crystallization of the *Wootz* of Western India with which they were manufactured (Journ. Royal As. Soc. No. VII.), and which would not be seen were they made with any other kind of steel. This proves that a trade must have existed between Damascus and Cutch; of which, indeed, there is other testimony. The best steel, in Pliny's time, came from China, that is, most probably from India. Steel was used in Egypt long before the Trojan war, when the Greeks, like the Peruvians at the time of the discovery of America, hardened their copper with an alloy of tin. A native sulphate of iron is found in the hills of Behar.

Copper being abundant in India, enabled the Hindoos to become acquainted with its ores, and make use of its preparations, both internally and externally. Lead is procurable in the form of galena in different parts of India, and has been obtained from Ava in the state of a natural litharge. The *Molybdæna* of the ancients is supposed by Dr. Thomson to be litharge, as it is described to have been in scales. Tin is one of the metals earliest known; it was employed by the Egyptians before the time of Moses, and is mentioned by the name *Bedel*, as procured, with iron and lead, from Tarshish. (Ezekiel, xxvii. 12). The Greeks and Romans obtained tin (*kassiteros*) from the Insulæ Cassiterides, or tin islands, lying off the north coast of Spain; hence it has been inferred that the Scilly Isles are intended, and that tin must always have been obtained from Spain or Cornwall. But the Hindoos, like the Egyptians, have employed tin for various purposes from very ancient times; and though there is no proof of its being found in the present day in the Peninsula of India, yet it is abundant on the opposite coast of the Bay of Bengal, as in Burma, Tenasserim, Junkseylon, and Malacca. There must in very ancient times have been a trade between India and these places. It is also found in the islands of Madagascar, of Banca, and Sumatra. Antimony, in the form of its sulphuret, was employed in remote antiquity, as in the present day by Asiatic females for painting the eyebrows and eyelids. It is the *stimmi* and *stibium* of the ancients, *itmud* and *ismud* of the Arabs, commonly known in India by the name *soorma*. With it, I believe, is frequently confounded the sulphuret of lead, which, in Northern India, is called *soormee* (*ee* is the feminine termination in Hindee) and used as a substitute for the former: a mistake, not of recent occurrence only, as Sprengel says, "Distinguit vero Plinius marem a femina." The sulphuret of antimony is produced in abundance in the island of Borneo; also, at Moulmein and in Pegu, in Persia, and in Caubul.

The ores of Zinc, calamine and blende, are produced in the province of Yunan in China, and it is said also in the Peninsula of India, and in Nepal. Until very recent times, zinc or spelter, was extensively imported from China into India. The name *tutenague*, by which Chinese zinc was known in commerce, is evidently derived from the Tamul, *tatanagum*. The common name, *tutty*, of impure oxide of zinc, is apparently also of eastern origin; as *tūtia* (Tamul *tootum*) is in common use in India and Persia, being applied to an ore of zinc imported from the latter. The sulphate of zinc is called *suffed* (white) *tutia*; sulphate of copper, *neela* (blue) *tutia*; and sulphate of iron, *hura* (green) *tutia*; so, in Avicenna, different kinds are described under this name, which occurs also in Geber. Of Arsenic, the Hindoos have been long acquainted with the white oxide, and the sulphurets. Of these, the first, or arsenious acid, called *sanchya* in Sanscrit, with Tamul, Hindee, and Malayan names, has been known in India from high antiquity, and imported from China; but it is probable, that it was also obtained artificially by the Hindoos. Realgar, or the red sulphuret, their *mansil* (Sans. *manahsila*), the *Sandaracha* of the ancients, is a product both of Burma and China, while the yellow sulphuret or orpiment (*Auripigmentum*) is so much a product of eastern countries, as to be imported into England even in the present day by its Hindee name *hartal* (Sans. *hartala*), being brought there from China and Sumatra: it is found also in Caubul and in Persia. The ores of arsenic and of mercury are, as far as hitherto ascertained, more abundantly found in China than in India, but as both are employed in medicine by the Hindoos, as well as by the Chinese, the fact, I think, indicates early communication between these nations. Chinese vermilion has long been famous; and, like native cinnabar from Japan, used to be imported into Europe. The Hindoos give processes for its manufacture, but it is also found in Tibet and in Nepal, and, according to Dr. Hamilton, occasionally also in Guzerat. Some other metals might be mentioned, as found within the limits we have been examining; as platina in Burma, manganese near Ajmere in Central India, and titanium in the Peninsula; but these not having been known as distinct substances to the Hindoos, it is needless to dwell longer on the subject.

As almost all the substances we have enumerated are also found in Europe, we might, as drawing inferences from the native countries of different substances, find it difficult, perhaps, to prove that their properties had not first been investigated in the West, and thence been communicated to the East. But the metals, we have seen were known in Egypt long before Europe was civilized, perhaps, even inhabited. From the same substances therefore existing both in the East and the West, we do not get any assistance from names, as European authors mention them of course only by their European names: yet, a few betray their origin, and leave little doubt that some at least, were first imported from the East. Thus, *misy* and *sory* of Dioscorides, have been shewn by Rossius, as quoted by Sprengel, to be Egyptian words, and both are supposed to be sulphurets of copper; but it is remarkable, that *mis* is a Persian name for copper, and that *missy* is a name frequently applied in India to sulphate of iron, of which the common Indian name, however, is *kusees*. Galen, in the prescription, transcribed at p. 79, expressly mentions *foreign misy* (*misyos peregrini* in the Latin translation).

Though Dioscorides has judiciously omitted taking any notice of the supposed medical properties of jewels and precious stones; yet as the majority of these are obtained from India, and were still more so in ancient times, so they corroborate the foregoing line of argument. They may be briefly enumerated, to complete the list of substances anciently used as medicines, and procured from India even in times as remote as those of the Persian Magi.

Thus, of siliceous minerals we have great variety of quartz crystals; amethyst, catseye, and calcedonies, as onyx, plasma, heliotrope, cornelians, and every coloured agate; with jaspers, in the island of Ceylon, in the rivers and mountains, as well of Central as of Peninsular India. Common garnets are found at great elevations in the Himalayas, but the precious variety with pyrope, in Ceylon and Pegu. From the former island we also have cinnamon-stone, with tabular spar; stilbite and heulandite from the Vindya, or transverse central range of Indian mountains, and Indianite with corundum from the Carnatic. So also, Ceylon and the opposite coast of Ava and Pegu, with the Capellen mountains, are equally famous for those ranked as aluminous minerals. Common corundum (Hind. *koorun*) has long been imported into Europe from Malabar and the Carnatic, where it occurs in granite rocks. Indeed, Dr. Thomson is of opinion, that the sand brought from the isle of Naxos and Ethiopia, which the ancients employed to facilitate the sawing of marble, was emery and corundum. So, also, in Ceylon and Pegu, are found the rhombohedral corundum or sapphire (*yakoot*), including the several varieties of blue or oriental sapphire (*H. nilam*); the red or oriental ruby (*H. manik*); and the yellow or oriental topaz (*H. pokhraj*); with the oriental emerald. The opalescent sapphire, with pearly reflections, is called *ayn-al-hireh*, or cat's-eye, in some Arabian works (Journ. As. Soc. Calc. 1. p. 353); but this must be distinguished from the common cat's-eye, the chatoyant variety of quartz. It is remarkable that the *Belioculus*, mentioned by Pliny, lib. 37. c. 55., is considered in the annotations by Hardouin, to be equivalent to *œil-de-chat*, and that this should be named in India *billi-ke-ankh*, or cat's-eye. In the above Arabic works, *turmali* (from which probably is derived our tourmaline (Singalese *tournamal*. Rees Cycl.), though applied by us to a different mineral v. Princep. l. c.) apparently embraces both the zircon and tourmaline families, as *turmali* is described as of a greenish yellow tinge, often called *zabarjad* or beryl; and specimens obtained in Calcutta proved to be the "jargoon of Ceylon," or precious zircon, which, when colourless, is cut and sold as a false diamond in the bazars of India. Here is also found the hyacinth zircon, with the topaz, chrysoberyl, and spinel ruby: the variety Balas ruby of the latter, occurs only near Balkh, in Badakshan. The emerald, it is supposed, was anciently procured from Upper Egypt only: less distinct varieties are now got from Cauganjam, in the Peninsular district of Coimbatore. The turquoise is produced only in the mines of Ansar, near Nishapore, in Khorasan; and, "in Badakhan, on the Jihun (Oxus) river, near where the Samarkand road crosses it, is the mine of *Lapis lazuli*." (J. A. S. 1. p. 362.) The other more common mineral substances found in the bazars of India, as *Serpentine*, *Soapstone*, &c., and many others, which are often mere varieties of one another, but have peculiar medical properties ascribed to each, are produced in various parts of the Primary and Trap formations of Central and Peninsular India. They will afford ample employment to those who, acquainted with the mineralogy of the country, and the names of the different substances in the various languages of the East, will endeavour to identify those said to be procured from India, of several of which native names are given in Pliny, lib. 37; as *sacal*, *sandaracus*, *sangenon*, *sacon*, &c. It would be interesting to ascertain, whether *Tabosheer* was known to the ancients, as it has from early times been employed in medicine by the Hindoos. The Arabic name is derived from Sans. *Twak-kshira*. The latter part of this compound is evidently the same as that mentioned in p. 36, as *syr.-diudar*, which Professor Wilson informs me is Sans. *khir*, *kshir* or *chir*, and means milk, milky juice or extract.*

In investigating the history of any subject among ancient nations, it is to be expected that the materials for inquiry will become fewer and more obscure, the higher we ascend. To this, as is well known, there is an exception in the accounts of India in the works of the ancients, for we find the references frequent, and the information both more original and correct, if we consult the works of the Greeks who wrote prior even to the time of Pliny and Galen.

* To do justice to the above subject of identifying the mineral, vegetable, and animal products, which were known to the Greeks and Romans, would require much more time and means than I at present possess; but it is hoped that others may be induced to pursue the subject. I regret that while these sheets are passing through the press, I have not had access to my own MSS., which may, perhaps, form the foundation of a future work on the Materia Medica of the East. In the mean time, I have been chiefly indebted for the various oriental names to the works of Carey, Roxburgh, and Ainslie, except where the obligations are separately acknowledged.

This is easily accounted for as a consequence of the increased communication of the Greeks with Persia and India, subsequent to the expedition of Alexander, the voyage of Nearchus, the reign of the Seleucidæ, and the embassy of Megasthenes and Onesicritus. In ascending, therefore, at once from Dioscorides to Theophrastus, or at least 300 years, it might be supposed, if we omitted taking the above facts into consideration, that the separation between these authors was too great to justify us in concluding that the same names always indicated the same substances, in these different times. To this, it may be replied, that though there were no celebrated authors during this period who treated expressly of the same subjects, yet there was throughout a series of writers on medicine, as well as of practitioners, who must have employed the same medicines; among which, those from the East always held a conspicuous place. Thus, Celsus, Archigenes, Andromachus, Aretæus, Cœlius Aurelianus, Soranus, Themison, Asclepiades, Heraclides, Serapion, Nicander, and many others lived during this time, and the sects of the Methodics, Pneumatics, and Eclectics, principally flourished. Hence it is most probable, that the knowledge of the names and drugs was correctly transmitted downwards. We may therefore safely infer, that the few drugs described even by Theophrastus, are the same as those which we find under the same names in Dioscorides: as, for instance, the two kinds of pepper, cinnamon, cassia, cardamoms, ebony, olibanum, costus, calamus aromaticus (καλαμος ευοσμος), schœnanthus, amomum, spikenard, and some others; with myrrh, crocus, carthamus, coriander, sesamum, &c. It is interesting to find that most of the above aromatic substances are described by Theophrastus (lib. ix. c. vii.), as being brought from India, with some from Arabia. Cinnamon and Cassia, I may mention, are described with

Comacum, which has not, I believe, been hitherto ascertained: but two kinds of it are described, one a fruit, and the other employed for mixing with the most precious ointments. This seems to me to be the substance of which we have only in recent times acquired any correct knowledge, and that is, the fruit of the cinnamon plant; and the fatty oil expressed from it, of which there are specimens in the College Museum of Materia Medica.

As Theophrastus treats of plants as a philosopher, and not with respect to their medical properties, many are necessarily omitted which must in his time have been well known. But for this very reason, several are particularly noticed, which are entirely overlooked by Dioscorides. These are frequently grouped according to general view as those which grow in mountains or in plains, wild o cultivated, &c., as well as such as are found in Africa, especially in Egypt; and with reference to our purpose it is interesting to find those enumerated which are peculiar to India.

Among these we find *Ficus indica*; and the plant, with leaves like those of the mulberry or vine (*Gossypium*), from which cloth is made, more particularly described as a produce of the island of Tylos, now Bahrein, in the Persian Gulf. Among the fruits also, is one remarkable for sweetness, serving as food for the Sapientes Indi, and of which one is enough for four men; the plant having long leaves, similar to ostrich feathers. Pliny, evidently describing the same plant, informs us, that its name is *pala*, though Arrian calls it *tala*. This there is little doubt must be the plantain (*Musa sapientum*), of which one bunch of the fruit frequently weighs many pounds; the long leaves also with their parallel veins at right angles to the midrib, becoming when blown about by the winds, divided into innumerable narrow shreds, justify the comparison to the feathers of the ostrich; and which, according to Garcias, "Nascitur etiam in Malavar, ubi *Palan* dicitur." (Clus. Exot. p. 229). The mangoe and tamarind are, perhaps, the other fruits, alluded to in the same chapter. The knowledge which had been attained is also observable in the accounts of the several grains cultivated in India; as rice, sorghum, the different kinds of millet, as of the use of some of the *Leguminosæ* and *Cucurbitaceæ*, for food.

Myrobalans having been so frequently referred to, it is necessary to observe, that the substances first known by this name, are not the same as those noticed at p. 36. The βαλανος or βαλανος μυρεψικη of Dioscorides, translated *Glans unguentaria*, celebrated in making the most precious ointments, is the *ban* of the Arabians, whence the *ben-nuts* of old writers, from which *oil of ben* was expressed. The seeds are those of *Moringa pterygosperma*, a native of India, as also of *M. aptera*, which is confined to Arabia and Egypt: the oil expressed from the seeds of both species is described as not becoming rancid; and being inodorous, is still employed in the East, especially for retaining the aroma of delicate flowers. Of the accuracy and minuteness of the information obtained in those early times, we have an instance in the passage of Pliny. lib. 12. c. 18. "Onesicritus tradit in Hyrcaniæ convallibus ficis similes esse arbores, quæ vocentur *occhi*, ex quibus defluat mel horis matutinis duabus." This plant has been supposed by Sprengel to be *Hedysarum Alhagi*, now *Alhagi maurorum*, from which the manna called *toorunjbeen* exudes; but from the form of the leaf it is much more likely to have been *Calotropis procera*, called *ashur*, or some nearly allied species: as on these also a kind of manna is secreted or deposited. Many other trees are mentioned; as being produced in India different from those in Greece, but which are stated to be without names.

The attention which was paid to the identification of plants, and the country in which they were produced, may be seen from the account given of the Ivy; which, though refusing to grow in some parts of Syria, was found flourishing in India on Mount Meru, the birth-place, according to some accounts, of Bacchus; this Harpalus attempted, but unsuccessfully, to cultivate in the gardens of Babylon. Bacchus is said also to have been the discoverer of the apple, and some other fruits, which are now found to be indigenous in the ramifications of Hindoo Khoosh,* where the holy Meru of the Hindoos is by the best authorities placed.

Considering, therefore, the minuteness and nature of the information obtained in those times, respecting even so remote a country as India; it is not assuming too much, or placing too great a reliance on our inferences, to conclude that a great portion of the substances mentioned as the produce of that country, are exactly the same as those, to which we now apply the names found in the early Greek authors. But this, according to the views we have taken, proves the still earlier investigation of their properties, and therefore the cultivation of medicine in the countries where alone these substances are found to grow. This will equally follow, even if it be denied that the several substances mentioned as Indian products, have been correctly ascertained; for there is no doubt that many such, whether correctly or only approximately ascertained, formed articles of commerce to, and were used as medicines in, the West, even in times prior to those of Theophrastus.

Admitting the above degree of knowledge of Indian plants and products at the time of the last-named philosopher, as subsequent to the Anabasis into Asia of Alexander; it might be contended that it afforded no proof of their having been known at any earlier period, as at that of Hippocrates, though he was anterior to Theophrastus only 150 years. The Father of Medicine is supposed to have lived 450 years before the Christian era; but so little is known of his history, that among his works are thought to be included many of those of his pupils and successors. Sprengel was of opinion, that they embraced altogether a period of 250 years, and that some were therefore subsequent to the time of Alexander, which he seems to assign as a reason for the knowledge displayed of Indian drugs; but anterior even to the time of Hippocrates, some of these were known in Egypt, through which channel it is probable they first became known to the Greeks.

Hippocrates is stated to have studied medicine under Herodicus, and to have embraced the philosophical hypothesis of Heraclitus; he is therefore classed among the followers of Pythagoras; and, like this philosopher, is described as having spent a considerable portion of his life in travelling in foreign countries, as Scythia, Colchis, Asia Minor, and perhaps Egypt, chiefly for the purpose of acquiring information, and studying the diversities of climate. Adopting the excellent abstract of Dr. Bostock, it appears that the philosophical tenets of Hippocrates were those of Heraclitus, "whose leading doctrine was, that fire is the prime origin of all matter, and that by the collision and peculiar combination of its particles, which are in perpetual motion, the four elements are produced. From this doctrine Hippocrates derived his leading principles of pathology, it lies at the foundation of all his medical hypotheses, and is brought forward in various parts of his works;" as "the body itself is supposed to consist of the four elements, combined in different proportions in different individuals:" and "the combination of the four elements into the four states or qualities with which they were affected, of hot, cold, moist and dry, gave rise to the four fluids or humours of the body; blood, phlegm, bile, and black bile, which originally tended to produce the four temperaments, and which, in their turn, contributed to the excess or defect of each of the humours." Hence arose the pathological doctrines, which, under the denomination of the Humoral Pathology, became the prevailing opinion of all sects and of all theorists, until the commencement of the eighteenth century. (Cycl. of Pract. Med. 1. p. xi). Dr. Bostock has, however, justly observed, that Hippocrates "appears to have had the sagacity to discover the great and fundamental truth, that in medicine, probably even more than in any other science, the basis of all our knowledge is the accurate observation of actual phenomena, and that the correct generalization of these phenomena should be the sole foundation of all our reasoning."

In examining the modes of applying remedies by Hippocrates as stated by Le Clerc, and the list of his Materia Medica, as given in the Index of Fœsius, the works of Sprengel and Dierbach, we find that he was indebted for it to the same sources as his successors, of whom, adopting the ascending series, we have already treated. Thus, with a great majority of European plants, we find the products of the Persian region, with drugs from Egypt, and spices and aromatics from India. Since mineral and metallic substances are mentioned chiefly for external exhibition, his Materia Medica consisted almost entirely of vegetable substances. These, it has been observed, from their being simply named in prescription, it is more difficult to determine, than where we have had their nature described; or find them arranged with similar products, as in the works of Theophrastus and Dioscorides. But as there is no reason to suppose that these authors applied the names found in

Hippocrates differently to himself, so do these, (as there is nothing contradictory in the medical properties ascribed to the several substances), indicate, with sufficient precision, the nature of the articles, as well as the countries whence they were procured.

As forming parts of a general system, which was probably more widely diffused than is generally supposed, it may be useful to enumerate the nature of the remedies, and the modes of applying them, which were adopted by Hippocrates. Like others of his contemporaries, the Father of Medicine appears to have been unacquainted with anatomy, and necessarily with physiology; but, like the Hindoos, he was remarkable for simplicity in prescription. He "was particular in watching the effect of external agents upon the system, such as temperature, the influence of the atmosphere, the effect of particular situations, the seasons, and other analogous circumstances;" and paid particular attention to diet, as well as to exercise, and prescribed baths, both general and local, as well as fumigations. He employed evacuations of various kinds as purgatives and emetics—"he prescribed diuretics and sudorifics; he drew blood both by the lancet and the scarificator; he applied the cupping-glasses; he administered injections and inserted issues; he made very frequent use of external applications, such as ointments, plaisters, liniments, &c." (v. Le Clerc and Bostock).

Of the articles of Materia Medica, for which Hippocrates was indebted to the Oriental or Persian region of botanists, we have Galbanum, Ammoniacum, Sagapenum and Assafœtida (if commentators are correct in considering Silphium to be this substance), Cummin, Coriander, Safflower, Saffron, and Scammony, with Sesamum. The pomegranate, and *Vitex Agnus Castus*, with some of the *Cucurbitaceæ*, and the oils called *Susinum* and *Narcissinum*, are all originally products of the same region, though it may be difficult to trace the course by which they were introduced into Europe. *Ricinus communis* was no doubt well known in Egypt; whence several other medicinal articles were procured, as we find them severally named Egyptian; as the so-called thorn and nut (probably *Hyperanthera aptera*); Ethiopian cummin (*Ptychotis copticum*, D.C., *P. ajowan* is given in India as this kind of cummin); so Egyptian salt, alum, earth, oil, and ointment, are all mentioned, as also a salt of Thebes.

Among the strictly Indian products, we have the two kinds of Pepper (long and round), Cardamoms and Ginger? (as this is probably what is called Ἰνδικον φαρμακον, v. Spreng. Hist. Rei. Herb. 1. p. 37); Cinnamon, Cassia, and Olibanum. Ebony is also mentioned, but this, and Olibanum, may likewise have been procured with Myrrh from Africa. *Amomum* not having yet been ascertained, need only be mentioned. The *Dolichos*, mentioned by Hippocrates and Theophrastus, as well as by later authors, is considered to be *Phaseolus vulgaris*, and to have been introduced from India in the time of Alexander. It is not found in the plains of that country, but is cultivated in Cashmere, whence I obtained seeds which vegetated in the Saharunpore Botanic Garden. *Nardos*, prescribed with Cinnamon and Myrrh, is probably the same substance as that described by Dioscorides, and therefore *Nardostachys Jatamansi* (v. p. 33); so *Cyperus*, *Schœnus* (σχοινος), and *Calamus* (καλαμος), are also enumerated with myrrh. The first may be the Indian variety of *Cyperus*, as we have shown, p. 37, that it is still used there as a perfume. Σχοινος, (Hippocr. ed. Fæs. sect. v. p. 574), mentioned also as σχοινου ανθος, sect. v. p. 665, and σχοινος ευοσμος, p. 673, with aromatics, is translated *Juncus odoratus*: this is considered by Sprengel to be *Andropogon Nardus*, but probably, more correctly by Dierbach *Andro-*

pogon Schœnanthus. The καλαμος enumerated with the above, sect. v. p. 574, mentioned as καλαμος μυρεψικος at p. 651, and translated *Calamus aromaticus*, is thought by Sprengel to be *Acorus Calamus*, v. p. 82, but is more likely to be *Andropogon Calamus Aromaticus* nob., v. p. 33, or some nearly allied species, as in later authors.

Among the saline, earthy, and metallic substances, we likewise find a number, which we have already noticed, as forming parts of Indian Materia Medica; but these it is sufficient merely to mention. Sulphur and bitumen, several earths and salts, as the loadstone, lime, nitre, and red nitre, with alum of different kinds, may have been obtained from Egypt and other parts of the world; together with lead, litharge, and cerusse, as well as copper, and its oxide in the form of scales. Iron with its oxides was also employed, as well as *misy*, v. p. 102; together with sulphuret of arsenic, both in the form of orpiment and of realgar.

Great as was the genius of Hippocrates, and admirably as it was suited, from the conjunction of powers of observation with those of generalisation, for investigating and advancing so complicated a science as medicine; there is no doubt that the full development of his mental faculties was owing in some measure to the impulse which had been given to philosophy and science during the preceding century, or from the time of Thales and Pythagoras. Previous to them, medicine is described by its historians (v. Le Clerc) as having been only an empirical art. But after reasoning had been introduced by these philosophers into the investigations respecting the phenomena of life, the powers and functions of the human body, and the causes and nature of disease; medicine began to assume the semblance of a science. These philosophers appear themselves only to have participated in the intellectual excitement which in those times pervaded all the civilized nations of the East. For the Persian Zoroaster is thought to have been born in the sixth century before the Christian era, and to have flourished in the reign of Darius Hystaspes. Confucius flourished in China in the same age, having been born, according to the best authorities, 550 B.C. While Buddhism, briefly characterised by Mr. Brian Hodgson as "monastic asceticism in morals, philosophical scepticism in religion," arose from the midst of Brahmanism in the plains of N.W. India (B C. 635), "in an age and country celebrated for its literature," where its doctrine and discipline became fixed by means of Sanscrit, one of the most perfect languages in the world, (Hodgson. J.R.A.S. 2. p.288), about the period when Nechao and the Pharaoh Hophra of Scripture reigned in Egypt. This was half a century previous to the very flourishing period of the Egyptian annals, or the reign of Amasis, who favoured the Greeks and allowed their traders to settle at Naucratis. It was during his reign, and about a century anterior to Herodotus, that Pythagoras is considered to have visited Egypt: but both were perhaps 1,000 years posterior to the most brilliant era of the rule of the Pharaohs. Subsequent to the time of Amasis, Grecian mercenaries were employed in the civil wars of Egypt: these afterwards settling in the country, it necessarily became inundated with Greeks.

Medicine is stated, by some authors, to have originated with the useful arts in Assyria, and by others in Egypt. In the latter, it appears to have been carried to the greater perfection, as may be inferred from its different branches having been practised by separate individuals, as well as from practitioners having been obliged to adhere to a written code. That the Greeks were originally indebted to this country is well known; but on this subject I prefer quoting the words of Dr. Bostock, who says, "It is generally admitted, that though Greece cultivated the arts and sciences with so much success, yet, in the first instance, she borrowed them from the neighbouring nations; principally, as it would appear, from Egypt, and, in some cases, from Phœnicia. To certain individuals, who migrated from these countries, the Greeks themselves were in the habit of referring the introduction of many of the most useful inventions; and during a considerable space of time, all those who were desirous of acquiring a larger share of knowledge, either theoretical or practical, than was possessed by their countrymen, visited Egypt, as the great storehouse of science and learning;" "so that in medicine, in the Orus and Thoth of the Egyptians, we may recognise the prototypes of the Apollo and Hermes of the Greeks."

Thales and Pythagoras are the Grecian philosophers who first visited Egypt. The latter, indeed, is described from his thirst for information to have travelled for a period of twenty-two years in Egypt, probably also Chaldæa, and some parts of Eastern Asia. Democritus is stated to have expended his patrimony in travelling, and to have been attached to medicine, as well as to other sciences. It is said, he visited Egypt, Persia, Babylonia, and India, where, according to Le Clerc, he had "des entretiens avec les philosophes, les géomètres, les médecins, les sacrificateurs, les magiciens, et les gymno-sophistes." (Hist. de Méd. p. 97). He is further described as having written on the nature of man; on pestilential diseases; on prognostics; on diet; on the causes of disease; on seeds, trees, fruits, and animals; and is mentioned by Pliny as also writing on the magical properties of plants; but among these, is an account of the "herbam æschynomonen, quoniam approprinquante manu folia contrahunt." This is no doubt the sensitive plant, which he could only have seen in southern latitudes.

Earlier than these times it is needless for our purpose to trace the history of medicine; but it presents a perfect blank from the Peloponnesian war to that of Troy, or for a period of about 700 years. It is interesting only to observe, that Podalirius and Machaon were sprung from Æsculapius, the god of physic, who is described as being the son of Apollo: in him we recognise not only the Orus of the Egyptians, but also the Surya of the Hindoos, as has been long ago (v. p. 57), remarked by Professor Wilson.

That Egypt was a highly civilized country, where philosophy and the sciences had, at an early period, made some progress, we might safely assume from its having been frequented by the Greeks for the purposes of study and information. That Lower Egypt was at a still earlier date a populous and flourishing kingdom; we know from the notice of it in Scripture, when visited by Abraham, about 1920 years before the Christian era. Memphis had at this time acquired great importance. The "hundred gated Thebes" is the constant theme of Homer's praise, and must have been founded centuries before his time (8 or 900 B.C.). Even this must be long posterior to the peopling and civilisation of Nubia, whence the tide of civilisation is concluded, on good grounds, to have descended along the banks of the Nile. For "Ethiopia's blameless race," who founded the ancient Meroë, and constructed the monuments of Nubia; must have flourished at a long anterior period. Because their temples, though similar to, are simpler than those, which, as the result of descending and improving ages, are, and ever have been, the wonder of ages. They were ancient also in the times, of what we now call those of ancient history. To have raised so many and such extensive structures,

Egypt must have been for many ages a thickly-peopled country; necessarily also, a richly-cultivated one. This indeed we know from history, where we often find it called "the granary of the world."

During much of this period, commercial intercourse, no doubt, existed between India and Egypt. But it is difficult to prove this, to the satisfaction of those, who do not allow the existence of eastern products in western markets to be sufficient evidence of the fact; or who deny that the substances mentioned in ancient writings, are identical with those to which we now apply the same names. The subject, however, has been so fully investigated and amply proved in the pages of Robertson and Vincent, as well as in those of the philosophical Heeren; that we have only to refer to their works, or make use of the materials which they have collected; to be assured that many of the substances we have found described in the oldest works on Materia Medica, constituted objects of a still more ancient commerce.

In examining the articles of this commerce, and the routes by which they reached the nations most distant from the countries where they were produced; it is difficult to determine where it is preferable to commence. But as some portion of the Persian empire, is generally supposed to have been the earliest peopled; and as the Hindoos point to the north as the direction whence they entered their present country, it will be preferable to trace the connexion between India and Persia, and between these and Babylon: the city of which there is the earliest historical and commercial record.

The early communications with India, as has been clearly shown by Heeren, were, as in the present day, both by land and by sea. The former is conceived to have taken place by Attock. We may picture to ourselves, caravans loaded with its natural and manufactured treasures, as proceeding from N.W. India, crossing the Indus at Attock, and proceeding along Caubul; where they were joined by the merchants from the mouths and from along the western bank of that river. From beyond Caubul, a branch turned, as in the modern day, towards the flourishing Bokhara, Samarcand, and Balkh, "the mother of cities." The main route continued west, though sometimes taking a circuitous direction to avoid deserts, or for the purpose of visiting flourishing districts; and passed near the modern Candahar, Herat, and through the Caspian Straits (Pylæ Caspiæ) to Ecbatana, the modern Hamadan. From this the caravans might either diverge southwards to Susa; or, crossing the long but direct communication, between this the capital, and the distant Sardis in Asia Minor, reach Babylon by continuing a nearly western course.

Babylon, even in the earliest times of which we have any notice, is mentioned as a populous and civilized city. Heeren has shown how admirably its position, at the head of the Persian Gulf, suited it, like so many other succeeding cities, for benefiting by the Indian trade. Communicating on the south by the Indian ocean with Arabia and India; and having the Euphrates extending to the north; by which it might hold intercourse with the nations between the Black and Caspian Seas on the one hand; and on the other with those on the shores of the Mediterranean. From Babylon, the merchant might thus proceed up the Euphrates or along its banks, into Armenia, or only as far as Circesium or Thapsacus; diverging from the latter into Syria; or from the former to the Phœnician colonies, by Palmyra in the Desert and Balbec in Cœlosyria.

These were cities said to have been founded by Solomon for the encouragement of this very traffic, of which the former extent is attested by their present ruins.

From Cœlosyria, the road led through Palestine into Lower Egypt. But both Palestine and Lower Egypt were probably more easily reached, by the caravans, led by nomad Arabian and Syrian tribes, from Gerria (a colony of Babylonians on the Persian Gulf) across the desert to the ancient Petra. Or, by that, which departing from Hadramaut and Saba, in Yemen, proceeded along the eastern coast of the Red Sea through Old Mecca and Leucocome, to the same Petra in Edom. This was one of the sites of commerce in the time of Alexander, probably also long before; its lately visited magnificent ruins, attest its former riches and flourishing state. To complete the course of the land communication, it may be stated, according to Heeren, that there was constant intercourse from Memphis to Thebes in Upper Egypt, and from that to Meroë in Ethiopia. These were all great marts and entrepôts for ancient commerce, and indebted to it alone, for their splendour and magnificence. Meroë communicated on the east through Axum with Saba and Adule on the western coast of the Arabian Gulf; while through Thebes, the caravans passed much further to the westward, as through Ammonium and Cyrene, even to Carthage and the interior of Africa.

Though it might be thought difficult, to bring proofs of all these routes, having been frequented in ancient times; nothing can be more satisfactory than the ingenuity with which Heeren has adduced passages from ancient authors, to explain the course of this commerce: which he considers also as a reason for the founding of so many flourishing cities in the midst of deserts. These we know have gone to ruin, chiefly since the Indian trade has taken flight from the Red Sea and Euphrates, to round the Cape of Good Hope. One quotation will be sufficient to prove that the products of the East reached Egypt by land-carriage in very remote antiquity. "In the 37th chapter of Genesis, it is related that the brethren of Joseph, when about to leave him to perish, saw a company of Ishmaelites, or Midianite merchants approach, to whom they resolved to sell their brother as a slave. Here Dr. Vincent well remarks: "upon opening the oldest history in the world, we find the Ishmaelites from Gilead conducting a caravan of camels loaded with the spices of India, the balsam and myrrh of Hadramaut, and in the regular course of their traffic, proceeding to Egypt for a market. The date of this transaction is more than seventeen centuries prior to the Christian era; and notwithstanding its antiquity, it has all the genuine features of a caravan crossing the desert at the present hour. (Prelim. Disq. to Transl. of Arrian's Periplus of the Erythræan Sea).

Some of the above routes terminating on the sea-coast, and at places formerly considered to produce articles, which we now know could only be obtained from India; clearly indicate that they must themselves have had communication by sea with that country. Of this, we have, unfortunately, but few accounts in early times; but how little do we know even now of what is very extensive; that is, the commercial relations of the Arabians with Africa and India. It has been observed by Dr. Vincent, that though there was extensive communication between Egypt and India, yet that neither the Hindoos nor the Egyptians were navigators enough to leave, though they made much use of, their own magnificent rivers. The Chinese seem to have been confined to their own seas and the East-India islands, and the Malays to between these and the coasts of the Continent of India; so that the carrying trade between India and Egypt must have been in the hands either of the Arabians or Phœnicians; and, according to the testimony of authors, appears to have been participated in by both. But it is not improbable that the Indians of Sinde may also have been among the early navigators, particularly as India not only afforded timber for the construction of ships; but its most ancient laws indicate an increased rate of interest for commercial adventures at sea.

The Phœnicians, however, are known to history as the great navigators of antiquity; who spread their colonies along the coasts of the Mediterranean, and carried their trade even to the shores of England and the north of Europe. Sidon is one of the most ancient cities of which we have any record, and it is supposed may have been founded as early as 2740 B.C. Sidon and Tyre were leagued together in the time of Moses. Their most brilliant period was from the time of David to that of Cyrus, or from 1000 to 550 B.C. The Phœnicians, though they had an establishment at Memphis, do not seem to have traded directly by sea with Egypt until the time of Amasis, when the ports were opened to strangers. But they were such skilful seamen, that they were employed in the reign of Necho in circumnavigating Africa. They were not freely admitted to the Red Sea, for the ports there were in the hands of the Edomites. But when the limits of Judea were extended thus far by King David; the Hebrews engaged in a maritime commerce with the Phœnicians; and their ships proceeded with those of Hiram, King of Tyre, from Elath and Eziongaber, at the head of the eastern gulf of the Red Sea, to Ophir and Tarshish.

As this participation in the Indian trade of the Red Sea, could not be continued after the Edomites had reconquered Elath and Eziongaber; the Phœnicians might be supposed to have enjoyed its advantages by sea for a comparatively short time. But Heeren has clearly shown, that long before the Persians had made themselves masters of Babylon, that is, B.C. 561; the Phœnicians had establishments for the pearl fishery and the Indian trade, on the isles of Tylos and Aradus, the modern Bahrein in the Persian gulf. The former existence of these is attested by the remains of their temples, and the prevalence of so many Phœnician names of places in the Persian gulf; as Aradus, Sidodona, and Szur or Tur near Cape Macate, mentioned by Nearchus as an entrepôt for Indian produce. From these Phœnician colonies, the Gerrians, (whose city is described as rich and populous), probably obtained Indian produce to despatch by caravans across the desert to Petra, or by water to Babylon. The vessels of the Persian gulf are considered by Heeren to have proceeded to Crocala, now Curachee at the mouth of the Indus, and Barygaza, now Baroach in the gulf of Cambay, and from thence even to the coast of Malabar and the island of Ceylon. As the Bahrein islands are supposed to be the Dedan of Scripture, so the passages in Ezekiel, xxvii. 19, 24, and xxxviii. 13, and of Isaiah, xxi. 13, 15, must be considered as applying to these voyages. (v. Heeren, On the Commerce of the Phœnicians and Babylonians).

But the Phœnicians did not enjoy the exclusive advantages of the maritime trade with India. For the Arabs also were great navigators; and always carried on an active commerce with the opposite coast of the Red Sea. Mr. Wilkinson considers that Old Kosayar was built as early as B.C. 1686 for the trade with Arabia; the other Egyptian ports along the same coast, as the Old Berenice, Adule, and Saba, were also frequented by the Arabs. The commerce between Meroë in Ethiopia, and Hadramaut and Yemen, especially from Adule to Aden, was, even, seven and eight centuries before the Christian era, in the most flourishing state. The communication from these to India, was much easier than can be conceived by those, accustomed only to the storms and uncertainties of northern seas; for there the monsoons blow with steadiness and regularity from autumn to spring from India to Africa, and from spring to autumn from Africa towards India. Thus wafted to its shores, there would be no difficulty in sailing along the pepper-yielding coast of Malabar, or to the cinnamon-producing Ceylon, which we know was the centre of an extensive commerce in later times. Even so early as the commencement of the Christian era, Pliny relates that an embassy was sent to the Emperor Claudius, who stated that the Cingalese traded as far as Serica; the Greeks had obtained very accurate accounts respecting this island in the time of the Seleucidæ; and extensive ruins of Hindoo-built temples remain in Java to attest its former connexion with India.

This active and extensive communication, both by land and sea in ancient times, indicates a great demand for the products of the country, which seems always to have been its ultimate object. But these were not to be obtained, without bringing materials for exchange, or gold and silver for purchase: since these valuable metals, though not wanting, were probably, at all times, more deficient than other substances, within the limits of the Indian territory. Thus the caravans obtained, in exchange for the products of India, those which were peculiar to the countries they visited; and which were of value, if not in India, at least in some part of the widely-spread regions, through which they passed. Thus, in Bactria and the Northern India of Herodotus and Ctesias, the modern Tartary and Tibet, they obtained gold and gold dust, probably also copper, lead, cinnabar, and tincal; still found in those regions. Furs may have been obtained from Siberia. Cattle appear to have been as numerous, and their wool as valuable, in ancient as in modern times. The woollen cloths, mentioned as so highly esteemed, were probably shawls from the wool of the Tibetan goat. The climate, though bleak, is abundantly supplied with grasses and leguminous plants, in the seasons when alone the country was visited by nomad tribes. The *Silphium* also is found in these regions; this may be either the Assafœtida plant, or the Prangos of Mr. Moorcroft, both belonging to the natural family of *Umbelliferæ*, and both fed on by cattle even in the present day. The country continues to be celebrated for its large dogs, which were formerly esteemed in Persia. Ctesias also mentions, that these Indians possess an insect, which affords a red colour found with *electrum* (resin?) on trees. From this it would appear, that the lac insect and resin were known, even in those early times. But there seems to be some confusion as to the country whence they were procured; for we cannot suppose that the same insect is found in the hottest parts of India, and the cold arid table land of Tartary. This mistake has perhaps arisen from their being, as we learn from Lieut. Burnes's Travels, a species of cochineal, found (like the scarlet-grain of Poland) on the roots of a plant, which flourishes in the marshes of Herat.

Persia, taken in the most extended sense, is celebrated both for salt deserts and fertile vales, hot plains and cool mountains. Hence it is possessed of a variety of grains, as well as of excellent fruits, with highly-valued gum-resins. The vine is well suited to the climate, as is the mulberry for the silk-worm, and the plains of Media for the *Medica herba* (clover), found also in Caubul. It was rich in metallic treasures, and still yields a great variety of useful products. Thus, its horses have long been celebrated; its long-tailed sheep yield a wool useful for some of their manufactures, as, for the carpets called Turkey, from their place of export to Europe; the goats of Kerman also yield a valuable wool. Copper is abundant in many parts of Persia, as in Muzanderan and Kerman. There were also mines of iron and of silver, which are now neglected. Still further north the metals were and are abundant in Caucasus, whence silver used to be obtained, as well as some gold. Maden, in the heart of Taurus, is celebrated for its mines; and is said to yield excellent copper, as well as some iron, silver, and gold. Copper and iron were known to the Masagetæ in the time of Herodotus. Xenophon mentions the numerous copper utensils among the Cadusii; and the Chalybi were early celebrated for their iron and steel. The saphire, found in Persia, is probably *Lapis lazuli*, which, as well as the turquoise, we have seen (p. 103), is abundant in Persia. The *Vasa murrhina*, said to have been made in Caramania, are considered by Dr. Thomson to have been formed of fluor spar.

Babylon, which, though long anterior to, may be considered as a portion of this empire; it owed its riches chiefly to its being an entrepôt for this extensive commerce. Without any trees but the cypress and the date, of which the fruit afforded food and its sap might be fermented into wine; the country was fertile only from the attention paid to irrigation in this warm climate. Its soil afforded clay for bricks, and calcareous concretions, as well as bitumen, for mortar. Cotton was cultivated in the island of Tylos, probably also in the neighbourhood of the capital; where it was no doubt weaved into cloth, and dyed of a variety of colours, constituting, according to some, the *sindon* of the ancients. Silk is likewise thought to have been weaved into cloth, and dyed of different colours. The Babylonians were likewise celebrated for the manufacture of scents, carved ornaments, and seal stones. Tylos furnished them also with timber and pearls.

The Phœnicians were indebted for their riches, to their commerce, which consisted chiefly of exchanges, and but little to the variety or extent of the products of their small territory. Manufacturing skill, however, enabled them to produce some articles, which were in the highest estimation; as the cloth of Sidon, and the purple of Tyre: with this were dyed both cotton, linen, and woollen cloths, as well as those of silk, according to some authorities. In addition to these, they manufactured glass, and made ornaments of various kinds. From Syria and Palestine they drew their corn, oil, and wine, as well as the wool of the desert. Their colonies along the Mediterranean yielded them the products of Africa, and of the south of Europe. Malta is said, to have grown and manufactured cottons: Elba afforded them iron. Spain contained their most distant, and at the same time most valuable settlements; itself yielding almost every thing that was peculiar to the others. Its warm climate in southern, and its cool in northern latitudes, enabled it to grow the grains and fruits of both tropical and European regions, and for these it has always been celebrated; also for its riches in oil and wine, and like all dry cool countries, for the fineness of its wool. Its mines yielded both tin and lead, also some gold and especially silver; the mines of the latter in the Sierra Morena were formerly rich and highly celebrated. The Phœnician commerce, however, extended beyond Spain: it reached even the Scilly Isles for tin and also lead, as well as the coast of Samland, in Prussia, for amber.

The foregoing enumeration, following only the course of what may be called the northern route, it remains to notice that, which embraced the more southern countries of the ancient world. This includes Egypt and India, with Arabia placed between them and forming a real entrepôt, both by position and by the Arabs having been the carriers of the produce of the far-famed East: as their countrymen in later times, served to transmit the sciences both of the West and of the East from ancient to modern times. Their country early acquired credit for abounding in spices, aromatics, and the most fragrant essences. Though Arabia possesses the horse, and the camel, emphatically called "the ship of the desert," enabling the Arabs to form caravans across their deserts; the country, examined by modern naturalists, as Niebuhr and Forskal, yields few products to justify the ancient commendations. *Balsamodendron gileadense*, the Balsam of Gilead-tree, like the Date Palm, was indigenous. Coffee was probably unknown, and Senna, as far as we know, unnoticed. Olibanum (*looban*, near Hadramaut. Niebuhr), Myrrh, and Aloes, may have been produced within its limits; but the largest quantities of both are now imported, chiefly into Aden, from the opposite coast of Africa. The Saumalees bringing down to the coast, from Cape Gardafui to near Bab-al-Mandel, Gum, Olibanum, and Myrrh, with other drugs, as well as Gold and Ivory, like the Macrobians of old. (Heeren.) Among the cultivated and wild, useful and ornamental plants, in the lists furnished by Forskal, we see no others which could have called forth encomiums, or become articles of commerce. Among them, we even find some American plants, as Tobacco, the Papaya, Anona, and others. Many of the fruits belonging to the family of *Rosaceæ* were probably introduced from Persia; and others, no doubt, from India, as the Tamarind (*tumr-hindee*, Indian date), Orange and Lemon, Mangoe (erroneously translated *Mangostien* in many works), the Plantain, Cocoa-Betel-nut and Fan Palms. Among the *Odores*, we have even Rue and Wormwood; with them also the Keura, which is, indeed, noted as affording one of the most fragrant essences. But this is the *Pandanus odoratissimus*, a truly Indian plant, often alluded to by Hindoo poets,* and having Indian names (Sans. *Ketukee*, Hind. *Ketgi* and *Keura*), the evident originals of that by which alone it is

* Through the air,
The slowly rising breezes spread around
The grateful fragrance of the *Ketaki*.
Wilson, Hindoo Theatre, II. p. 85.

known. The Ginger, Zedoary? (*Curcuma rotunda*) Ricinus, Sesamum, Cotton and Sugar-cane, are equally Indian. *Saj*, *Abnoos*, and *Shishum*, that is, Teak,* Ebony, and Sissoo (*Dalbergia Sissoo*), are expressly mentioned as *woods brought from India*. (v. Forskal. Flora Ægypto—Arab. p. xcvi.) From identity in latitude, and similarity in climate, with some parts of India, there is no doubt also a resemblance in the Botany of the coast of Arabia, in the families of *Cucurbitaceæ*, *Leguminosæ*, and *Gramineæ*, as also in some others: but there is a total absence of a great proportion of the substances, which were thought by the ancients to be produced in Arabia.

Egypt is well known as having always been fruitful in corn, and famous for its manufacture of linen cloth; which must have formed its principal articles of export to Arabia, Phœnicia, and Abyssinia. It has also been famed for its emeralds, sometimes confounded with simple fluor spar. Gold was early extracted from its mines, as well as received, with ebony and ivory, in tribute from Ethiopia. Silver was less common. Recently both copper and iron mines have been discovered in the hills between Egypt and the Red Sea, but lead only in the neighbourhood of Mount Sinai. Tin has nowhere been found. Besides emeralds, the topaz, amethyst, lapis-lazuli, and alabaster, as well as sulphur and petroleum, have been found in Egypt or the islands of the Red Sea.

Among the vegetable products of Egypt, we find variety as well as abundance for the support of its numerous population; with two annual crops, dependent on irrigation

* Some of the Persian authors consider *Saj* to be the *Sal*, *Shorea robusta*, also a valuable and much-used timber-tree; but as the Teak is the best known, and most highly valued timber-tree on the Malabar coast; and as the *Saj* is described, in the same Persian works translated from the Arabic, as having large leaves like elephant's ears: it is evident to those acquainted with both trees, that this can apply only to those of *Tectona grandis*.

and on the overflowing of the Nile. The separate substances are almost all the same as those cultivated in India; of Mr. Wilkinson's list, the Clover, Lupin, and Dyer's Madder, are the only plants which are not so. The roots and seeds of three kinds of Lotus (*Nelumbium speciosum* and two *Nymphæas*) also afforded them food. The Vine extensively cultivated, yielded wine; and the Olive, oil; the Date-Palm, both food and an article of export to the Arabs and Africans. The Peach was probably introduced from Persia. The plant called *Persea*, has been supposed by different botanists to be either *Balanites ægyptiaca*, or *Cordia Myxa*, both of which are Indian plants; the former is also common in the deserts of Egypt: but neither appears to me to agree with the descriptions of the fruit of *Persea*. The Cotton, though introduced in later, does not seem to have been known in the early times of Egypt; for it is never found in their tombs, the cloths investing mummies having been ascertained, by microscopic observation, to be invariably linen. But among the substances the produce of Egypt, as among those of Arabia, we do not find either spices or aromatics, or even perfumes. The flowers of Egyptian plants are, indeed, expressly mentioned as being without scent. Neither do we find any of the substances which they required for their sacrifices, or for the purposes of embalming; these, therefore, they must have procured by commerce with a distant, though still the nearest country, India and its pendent Ceylon.

From the absence, therefore, of such substances from the soil of Egypt, and their presence in the arts and religious ceremonies of its inhabitants; we might, independent of other testimony, deduce a commercial connexion with countries however distant, which were alone capable of supplying such articles. Hence we should be led to infer an intercourse between Ancient Egypt and the probably equally Ancient India. This is authenticated by the presence of Indian plants in the former: thus, the Cotton, which is truly such, though absent in the earliest, was no doubt known in later times, as some of the seeds have been found by Rosselini in one of the tombs at Thebes. So also, *Nelumbium speciosum*, the far-famed Lotus; though it has now disappeared from, was formerly as highly esteemed in Egypt, as it has ever been in its native country, India: where still prevails the practice of sowing its seeds by rolling them up in a ball of clay, as is described to have been the usage in Egypt. Its roots, stalks, and seeds, as well as those of species of *Nymphæa*, afford articles of diet to the Hindoos of the present day, as they did to the Egyptians of old. Other plants might be similarly adduced, as well as the absence of those, of which the products appear to have been in use in Egypt. "On reconnâit meme, à ce que nous assure Denon, des bois de l' Inde dans les sièges et autres meubles." Heeren vi. p. 158. Fr. ed. So Rosselini informs us, that there is an Egyptian harp at Florence, of which the wood is what is commonly called East-Indian mahogany. (Athenæum, 22d July, 1837). This may be *Cedrela Toona*, or some of the woods mentioned at p. 128, as imported even in our own day from India into Arabia.

It may, in addition, be useful, to note some other points in which there is a similarity between the two nations. Thus the arts practised by both, are very similar, not only in nature, but also in many of the processes which they adopt. Agriculture, with the modes of irrigation, is one of these; but being dependent in a great measure upon climate, may appear less striking. Weaving, Embroidering, Dyeing, Glass-making, and Working in Metals, seem to have been commonly practised in both. Flax or linen was, no doubt, a very early manufacture in Egypt, but the representations on their temples of the transparent fabrics, emphatically called "woven air," forcibly recal to mind the finest muslins of India. Dr. Thomson (Hist. of Chemistry) has adduced the remarkable passage of Pliny, lib. xxxv. c. 11, to show that the Egyptians were acquainted with a process very similar to Calico-printing, an art which the Hindoos have practised from time immemorial.

Architecture, however, is the art which has most generally been acknowledged, and naturally so, from its conspicuous nature, to be that in which the resemblance is most striking. The peculiar style, and the colossal dimensions of the cave-built temples of Upper Egypt, bear so strong a resemblance to those of Elephanta, Salsette, and Ellora, in Western and Peninsular India; as to have induced many authors to ascribe a common origin to nations, which, in the earliest ages, and at such distances from each other, produced such similar structures. The very same mode of quarrying great blocks of stone by means of fire, and apparently the same mode of polishing the hardest rocks, was practised by the one, as it now is by the other. So similar is some of the architecture of the two countries, that the recent work on "Egyptian Antiquities," has a special chapter on Indian temples. This similarity is also seen in the peculiar mode of making arches, common to the two countries,* and likewise in the varied design and

* In the observations on the old Temple of Vishveshwur, in Prinsep's Views of Benares, it is stated that the domes of Hindoo temples, built after ancient models, are not formed on the principle of the arch, but by successive protrusion of the courses of stone, and by cutting off the angles laterally, so as to change the square into a polygon, and thence gradually into a circle. The same may, I think, be seen in the ancient Hindoo temple in the fort of Adjighur, as well as, I believe, in the fort of Kallinjer, where gigantic sculpture and cave-built temples on a small scale are also conspicuous. So "we find in Egypt, ancient arches of stone, constructed, not as ours, with

ornaments of different pillars in the same colonnade.* The resemblance, in the colossal sculpture and general appearance of the deities in the two countries, has also been frequently remarked. So striking was it to the Hindoo soldiers, who accompanied the expedition from India, that, scrupulous as they usually are, they did not hesitate to perform their devotions in the temples of Egypt, on recognising the characteristics of their own places of worship. (Heeren. vi. p. 186. French edit.) The Sphinx is also found in India as in Egypt. (v. Eg. Antiq. 1. p. 125.) So also, at Naga, in the desert of Upper Nubia, south of Meroë, and to the east of the Nile: on one of the most ancient monuments, the god Ammon is seen in one place with the lion's head and ram's horns; and in another, with two heads and four arms; which Heeren remarks, is the only representation he is acquainted with in Egypt, which reminds us of Indian combinations. (Heeren. v. 133. Eg. Antiq. 1. 171.)

If we have hitherto drawn an argument from the prevalence in these two countries of similar arts; we may also draw an inference from the absence in both of others,

with a key-stone, but by placing the stones in horizontal layers, in such positions and proportions, that the parts which are over a gateway or entrance, are in no danger of falling in; the upper and irregular stones of the doorway are then chiselled into a circular curve, which has all the appearance of an arch without really being one." (Eg. Antiq. 1. p. 209.) Crude brick arches were, however, in use in Egypt about 1540 B.C. (v. Wilkinson's Thebes, p. 510.) "But Strabo and Herodotus agree in saying, that the Indian caverns or excavations were justly presumed to be more ancient than the temples of Egypt." (Hoskings on Architecture. Encyc. Britt. 7th Ed.)

* These may be distinctly seen in the ancient Hindoo colonnade, near the foot of the Kootub Minar, near Delhi. The Mahomedans, instead of mutilating the columns, fortunately only concealed the numerous carved figures and rich decorations, with plaster. This was carefully picked out by Lieut.-Colonel Smith of the Bengal engineers, when employed by the Indian Government in repairing the Kootub Minar.

especially that of coining money; which seems to have been unknown in Egypt, as it was in India until after the reign of the Seleucidæ. The earliest Egyptian money is described as having been in rings, which were weighed when used as instruments of exchange.

In addition to the arts, we may adduce some of the sciences as equally cultivated both by the Egyptians and by the Indians; though the former are not supposed ever to have attained the same degree of proficiency as the latter. Thus, Geometry, in some degree Astronomy, which afterwards degenerated into Astrology, Music, and Medicine, were all cultivated by the Egyptians. Their medicine is said by some to have consisted only in the practice of magical arts; notwithstanding that the Greeks adopted many of their more efficient remedies. The degree of proficiency attained by them in each of the above sciences, is not easy, if at all possible for us now to ascertain.

Besides the above arts and sciences, and perhaps still better calculated to show the resemblance between the ancient Egyptians and the present Hindoos; is the physiognomy, dress, and the representation of the different arts as practised by the former, and figured on their monuments. So great, indeed, is this resemblance, that it is hardly exaggeration to say, that they might be introduced into a book of modern travels, as representations of Hindoo artisans. As geologists from observation of recent phenomena, infer what must have occurred in the primeval ages of the world, so might we from investigating the processes of the arts as at present practised by the Hindoos; better understand the hints and descriptions in ancient authors, as well as the representations on ancient monuments, of those practised by the Egyptians. Their division, moreover, into castes, especially into the military and priesthood, as well as the similarity in their divinities (v. Sir Wm.

Jones on the Gods of Italy, Greece, and India), their religious belief, and that in the metempsychosis, are all points of coincidence, which we cannot believe to be accidental.

That it was not so, we know from the relations of ancient historians; Herodotus and Diodorus Siculus, as quoted by Heeren, state that the Pharaohs were conquerors, as well in Ethiopia as in Bactria and India. Xenophon, in the Cyropædia, mentions alliances between the people and states, from the banks of the Nile to those of the Oxus, Indus, and Ganges. The paintings on the monuments of Thebes are considered to refer to wars in Assyria, Bactria, and India: as, Indians, and also Asiatic Ethiopians, or at least some southern Asiatic nation, are depicted on the palace of Osymandyas and at Medinet-Abou. The great river or sea, which is always introduced, is supposed to be the Euphrates: it may be the Indus, or the gulf of Persia, or perhaps some part of the Indian ocean, as Sesostris is described as having conquered some Indian islands (v. Heeren. vi. p. 235-317). That Indians were sometimes the aggressors is apparent from a quotation made by Heeren from Syncellus, p. 120. ed Venet. which he translates, "Æthiopes, ab Indo fluvio profecti, supra Ægyptum sedem sibi eligerunt," stating that as this was during the most brilliant period of Thebes, in the reign of Amenophis the Memnon of the 18th dynasty, B.C. 1430, they could not have given origin to the people, nor to their civilization. Sir Wm. Jones on the contrary mentions, that he is "strongly inclined to believe that Egyptian priests have actually come from the Nile to the Ganga and Yamuna (Ganges and Jumna), which the Brahmans most assuredly would never have left. They might, indeed, have come either to be instructed or to instruct; but it seems more probable that they visited the Sarmans of India, as the sages of Greece visited them, rather to acquire, than to impart, knowledge: nor is it likely that the self-sufficient Brahmans would have received them as their preceptors." (' Jones On the Gods of Greece, India, &c.')

Considering, that the resemblance between the Indians and Egyptians extends to so many points, it will be useful to indicate a few dates in the history of the latter, for the purpose of future comparison. The commercial intercourse between the two countries is well known to have been most active, subsequent to the reign of the Ptolemies; especially after Alexandria had been founded expressly for its encouragement. Previous to this, Egypt had been conquered by the Persian Cambyses, B.C. 525, and by the Kings of Meroë about 800 B.C.; from which to about 700 B.C. is considered the most flourishing period of the Ethiopian, but from the former to B.C. 1600, that of the Egyptian kingdom. This was during the reign of the 18th to the 23d dynasty of Diospolitans from Thebes, or that of the Sesostridæ, of whom Rameses the Great, the Sesostris of Herodotus, was the most distinguished. During this period the principal edifices are supposed to have been erected, and the Israelites to have departed from Egypt B.C. 1491, or 430 years after the arrival of Abraham. The Hyksos, or Shepherd Kings, who conquered and held possession of Lower Egypt from about 1800 to 1600 B.C., are supposed, by some authors, to have been an Arabian, and by others a still more eastern Asiatic (the Pali) race.

India seems, in the remotest antiquity, to have been famed for the variety and richness of its peculiar products; nothing, indeed, can be so strong a proof of their value, or of the great antiquity of the people, than finding even when the position of the country was unknown, that its products were familiar to, and desired by, all the most ancient and civilized nations of antiquity. These must have sought for them in their native countries; because we never hear of Hindoos travelling, either for information or for commerce, beyond the precincts of their own territory. There was little indeed to tempt them beyond, having every thing within their own limits; whether food, raiment, or the means of cultivating the different arts; with a fruitful soil and favourable climate, for the development of the physical and mental resources of a resident people.

The earliest known products of India have been so frequently mentioned, that we need not again recur to those which were known to the Greeks; except to repeat that their nature indicates the southern latitudes from which they were brought. That these were the shores of the Indian Peninsula, we may infer from their being the nearest tropical country where such products could be grown; Africa being then, as now, equally inaccessible both by land and by sea. India, therefore, independent of all other evidence, was, most probably, the ultimate object of the long journeys and voyages of antiquity. The occurrence of these we might indeed consider proved, by finding the products of the east and south, well known to and esteemed in the west, even though we were unable to trace the routes by which they reached their destination.

The fertility of the Indian soil, and the variety of its products, afforded not only ease and abundance to its inhabitants, but also leisure for other pursuits than that of procuring food. The north-western provinces, or those along the banks of the Ganges, were early seats of the highest civilization, and they enjoy particular advantages of climate. From October to March they are able to cultivate wheat and barley, with the pulses of Europe; and with equal success, in the rainy season, or from the middle of June to the end of September, rice, sorghum, and other tropical grains and pulses. Even in the hottest season, or from April to June, the *Cucurbitaceæ*, and some vegetables, may be cultivated by means of irrigation. The great variety of fruits also, as the plantain, jack, mangoe, with the several fecula-yielding roots, would serve not only as luxuries, but also as food.

The cotton, an indigenous and peculiar product, afforded clothing for its inhabitants. Silk, there is reason to suppose (v. Sir W. Jones), was early made use of. Several species of silk-worms are indigenous in the eastern provinces of India. (v. J. Asiat. Soc. vi. p. 21). Wool, and its valued manufacture, the shawl, were known at an early period, as the Persian name is said to be derived from the Sanscrit. The woods, minerals, and metals, afforded materials for numerous arts, as did the various vegetable colours for dyeing; with ligneous fibre, gums, resins, oils, and natural varnishes. But many of the above substances, excepting, of course, the silk and cotton fabrics, being such as are found, or substitutes for them, in other countries, were not likely to have offered to distant nations, sufficient inducements to visit India or its shores.

But India had abundance of products, both peculiar and precious, and requiring only to be known to be highly valued. Among these its aromatics, such as cinnamon and cassia, were conspicuous. The spices probably included pepper and cardamoms, perhaps also ginger; while, among its perfumes, we have the sweet calamus, onycha, nard, and lign-aloe. The attr of roses we do not find distinctly noticed in the earliest periods; but pearls and precious stones formed very early articles of commerce; while indigo seems to have been detected in the blue stripes of some Egyptian mummy-cloths:—we know that, in later times it is mentioned as an article of export from India to Egypt (v. Egypt. Antiq. ii. p. 190.). Ivory and ebony were always abundant, and other woods may have been articles of export in ancient, as they are even in modern times to Arabia. The metals probably had their properties, as in the case of steel, first investigated in India; and were then sought for, and found, in countries which first procured them from a distance.*

The antiquity of the commerce of Indian products is, however, incontestably proved from our finding, even in the earliest records we possess, mention of the spices and aromatics, the precious stones, and probably also the cotton, wood, and metals of the East; a term in which India must be included, as the names of some of the substances mentioned appear to be derived from eastern sources, and often from the Sanscrit language.

Though in the earliest chapters of the books of Moses, we read of the working in metals, this probably alludes to gold, silver, and copper, all common in the ancient world, and easily worked, as well as iron, when found in sand or in a magnetic state. But silver, iron, tin, and lead, are described in

* The above view of the natural fertility, richness, and variety of the products of India, may strike many as contradicted by the fact of these being now chiefly noted for their inferiority, when they come into competition with those of other parts of the world, where similar products are grown. "This, it strikes me, was owing to the early cultivation of the mind, and the advancement of science among the Hindoos, which must have greatly influenced agriculture, as well as all the other arts of life. Since then, if India has not retrograded, she has certainly remained stationary, while the rest of the world has been advancing, and applying every fresh acquisition in science to the improvement of the varied arts and manufactures of civilized life." Conceiving it perfectly feasible, by the application of principles to practice, and by the adoption of other means suited to the end in view, to give an impulse to the improvement and multiplication of the products, and consequently to the resources of India, I was induced, in conjunction with the Right Hon. Holt Mackenzie, formerly Territorial Secretary to the Indian Government, and lately a member of the Board of Control, to offer some suggestions, and write a paper on this subject, which is printed in the Proceedings of the Royal Asiatic Society, 19th March, 1836.

Ezekiel, xxvii. 12, as being imported from Tarshish; and this word is by some authors supposed to be a Sanscrit compound, *tar-desa*, or silver country. Lead is thought by Bohlen to derive its Greek name *μολυβος* or *μολυβδος*, from *mulwa*, one of the names of lead, from the Indian province Malwa, whence it was procured. (Ægypt. Antiq. ii. p. 327.) Iron and steel are so ancient as Indian products, that it is difficult to trace them to their highest antiquity. Tin, we have shown, is abundant in the Malayan Peninsula. Antimony (*cohal* and *surma*) for painting the eyes, was anciently so employed, but is not peculiarly an Indian product. The word *chasmal*, translated *amber*, is thought to be a metallic substance, of which the nature is not well understood: "Out of the midst thereof as the colour of amber, out of the midst of the fire" (Ezek. 1. 4); is supposed not likely to be the substance now so called, also a product of India. It may, perhaps, be glass, as this was known to the Egyptians and Phœnicians at an earlier period. The word *chushm*, in the Arabic dictionary, is applied only to the eye.

The various precious stones, though frequently mentioned, being so difficult to identify, do not enable us to prove that they were procured from India; but we may infer from their abundance, that they were so, with the substances which could only have been brought from that country.

The Nitre of Scripture (Heb. *nether*) is probably only *natron;* and the soap (*borith*) thought by some to be borax, is, perhaps, some alkaline plant used for washing, and of which there are several on the coasts of the Red Sea: *Suæda* (soda) *monoica* of Forskal, is usually quoted. (v. Harris.) Sulphur (Heb. *gophreth*) is *kubreet* in Arabic, but *gunduk* in Hindee; while pitch, naphtha, and petroleum, are not strictly Indian products. *Copher* is by some thought to have reference to camphor, but this substance does not seem to have been known even in later times. It is probably more correctly translated the cyprus (κυπρος) of the ancients, which is the *henna* or *Lawsonia inermis*, extensively used by Asiatic women for staining their fingers and feet of an orange colour; and by the men their beards, previous to dyeing them black.

Some substances clearly indicate the trade carried on in ancient times: thus, *Galbanum* (Hebr. *chelbenah*) was probably obtained from Persia; so, the Balsam-tree (Hebr. *baalshemen*) though cultivated in Judea, was no doubt originally introduced from Arabia; while Myrrh (*mur*) must have been imported partly from Arabia, but also from the opposite coast of Africa. Frankincense or Olibanum (Hebr. *lebonah*, Arab. *looban*), is found both in Africa and India. The Fitches (*ketsach*), thought to be the seed of *Nigella sativa*, continue, like the Cummin (Hebr. *cammon*), with which they are mentioned, to be employed as condiments in the East.

The Gopher Wood of Scripture is so differently translated by different commentators, that it is difficult to form even a conjecture on the subject; besides being used at so early a time, and mentioned only once. It need not have been alluded to, except that the Arabic version translates it *saj*, which is the teak, and not likely to have been the wood employed. The Ebony (*hobnim*) may have been the Indian *abnoos*, but it was also obtained from Ethiopia.

The *Shittim-wood* is generally supposed to be the *black Acacia*, or one of those growing in Upper Egypt, which attain considerable size; as *Acacia vera*, *nilotica*, *Seyal*, and *tortilis*. But the word (*shittim*) is remarkable for its resemblance to the Sanscrit *shishum*, which is also that of a dark-coloured and most valuable wood, imported from India into Arabia even in the present day (v. p. 128).

The Algum or Almug-wood of Scripture may be the African *Thuya articulata;* but we have no clue to its identification, except that of its country, which is described as being *Ophir*, whence it was brought in plenty, with precious stones. (1 Kings. x. 11.) *Thuya articulata*, or the *Arar* tree of Barbary, yielding Sandarach, attains considerable size, and is much used, Dr. Lindley informs me, in the construction of mosques.

If there be some uncertainty respecting the country of some of the preceding articles, there can be none about those which follow, as they are, and ever have been, the produce of India. Among these we read frequently of spices, certainly an indefinite term, but usually considered as referring to the caravan trade, bringing the pepper of India, with cardamoms, and perhaps ginger, all found in abundance, and of excellent quality, on the Malabar coast. Cinnamon (Hebr. *kinnemon*) there can be no doubt about, as the name appears derived, like the Greek, from the Malayan or Cingalese appellation (v. p. 84.), as it is stated by Herodotus to be so called by the Phœnicians, and said to grow in the country where Bacchus was educated.* Cassia (Hebr. *kiddah*) is similarly Indian.

Spikenard (Hebr. *nard*) is most probably the perfume which was called *nardos* by the Greeks, and which we have seen, is *Nardostachys Jatamansi*, still employed in

* The author of the work, entitled "The Hindoos, &c." L. E. K., in stating "that some writers have been led by the similarity in sound of the names *Bâghês* and *Bacchus*, to assume the identity of the Hindoo and the Greek deity so called, and have considered the present worship of Mahadeva or *Bâghês* in these regions, as a confirmation of the supposed expedition of Bacchus into India," adds that "it should, however, be observed, that the similarity of the names *Bacchus* and *Bâghês* is but accidental; the latter word is a modern vernacular corruption of the ancient *Vyaghresa*, which is a compound of *Vyâghra*, "a tiger," and *isa*, "a master or lord." But is this not, rather a further confirmation, as Bacchus is represented as drawn in his chariot by a tiger and a lion; and that tigers, panthers, and lynxes, are described as following him in his Indian journey.

India in making a fragrant ointment, highly valued by the natives of that country. In connexion with this, may be mentioned the sweet Calamus, literally sweet cane or reed, (Exod. xxx. 23) where it is mentioned as one of the ingredients of the holy anointing oil; and in "the Spikenard and Saffron, Calamus and Cinnamon," Cantic. iv. 14; so, in Ezekiel, xxvii. 19, "bright iron, cassia and calamus, were in thy market;" and "to what purpose cometh there to me incense from Sheba, and the sweet cane from a far country," Jerem. vi. 20. In all these places, the word employed in the Hebrew is *kaneh-bosem*, which is translated sweet cane or calamus, and commonly thought to be equivalent to the *Calamus aromaticus* of the ancients. This, the καλαμος and καλαμος ευοσμος of the Greeks, is often stated to be the *Acorus Calamus* of botanists, a plant common in ditches and marshy parts of Europe, and in moist situations on mountains in India. It has a warm and aromatic taste, with some degree of aroma, but certainly too little, to have ever been thought worthy of being an article of commerce from distant countries; particularly as it might so much more easily have been found at home. The author of the notes on Exod. xxx. 23. in the Pictorial Bible, "apprehends that it was a species of *Cyperus*, since, &c. we know that several members of that genus have odoriferous roots, and are used as perfumes by the natives of the regions where they grow." (v. p. 83.) This most probably is much nearer it than the *Acorus Calamus*.

Having shown that the *Calamus Aromaticus* of Dioscorides (p. 33) is a species of *Andropogon* (a conclusion which had also been come to by Sprengel and Dierbach, with respect to the καλαμος ευοσμος of Hippocrates); I am of opinion that the Calamus of Scripture is the *Andropogon Calamus Aromaticus*, which I have mentioned at p. 33 and 113. This, for the delightful fragrance of its distilled oil, is more fully entitled to the commendations the *sweet cane* has received, and to have been sought for as an article of commerce from distant countries, than any other substance with which I am acquainted, the *attr* of roses hardly excepted. Of this any one may be convinced, by examining the specimen of this essence, which I have placed in the Museum of Materia Medica. I know not whether it be an accidental circumstance that the aromatic species of *Andropogon*, common in North-western India, instead of having a simple name like most other substances, is always designated by a compound term, *mirchia-gund* and *gund-bel;* so, in Hebrew, *kaneh-bosem;* in Greek, *καλαμος ευοςμος*; which I suppose to be *Andropogon Calamus Aromaticus*, nob. That a grass similar to the fragrant *Andropogon*, or at least one growing in the same kind of soil and climate, was employed by the ancients, we have the assurance, in the Phœnicians who accompanied Alexander in his march across the arid country of Gedrosia, having recognized and loaded their cattle with it, as one of the perfumes of commerce. It is in a similar country, that is, the arid plains of Central India, that the *Andropogon Calamus Aromaticus*, nob., is found, and where the fragrant essential oil is distilled from its leaves, culms, and roots. In consequence of Arrian using the word *nard*, Mr. Hatchett, who also considers this oil to be the precious ointment of Scripture, was led to suppose the plant to be the *nardos* of the Greeks; but it is not possible that this, so fully described by Dioscorides, can grow in the deserts of Kerman; as all the species are found only on the mountains of Europe, or on those of India, round which, according to Dioscorides, the Ganges flows. (v. p. 33.)

The Lign-aloe (Hebr. *ahalim*) I believe to be the *Agallochum* or Eagle-wood, mentioned at p. 88. Sir Wm. Jones also supposes, that " the fragrant wood called *Alluwwa* in Arabic, and *Aguru* in Sanscrit, must have been one of the early articles of commerce to the Western world." Another perfume of the East, which seems to have been early known, and is still employed, is the *Onycha* (Hebr. *shecheleth*) mentioned with Galbanum and Frankincense. This, by some commentators, is supposed to be *Gum Ladanum*, from the Arabic version; but it is much more probably, as its name indicates, the article mentioned at p. 95, as *Unguis odoratus*, and of which the Sanscrit name *nakhi*, is literally the same as the Greek *ονυξ*. This, according to Rumphius, who describes ten kinds of the odoriferous onyx, which serve as the basis the principal perfumes in the Indian islands, (Herb. Amb. ii. c. 17) is the operculum or lid of the shells of *Purpura* and *Murex*. This being flat, and something like a nail, explains the origin of its name: we may easily suppose it was brought with the other Indian substances to Egypt, Palestine, and Greece.

If the term *skukur*, so frequently employed in Scripture, translated strong drink, and always coupled with wine, be, as Dr. Harris suggests, and as is probable, wine and sugar, we have another Indian manufactured produce, early known in the West, as was also indigo, both noticed by Sir Wm. Jones as most ancient products.

The materials for clothing next require our attention. Egypt was always famed for its cultivation of flax, and manufacture of fine linen. Silk was probably known, as the word *serikoth* is employed in Isaiah, xix. 9, and is thought to be the origin of the Latin *sericum*, from *Seres*, whence the Greeks and Romans first obtained their silk.

Cotton, though undoubtedly known at a very early period in the West, has caused considerable debate. This is owing to several different words being used in the Hebrew text, which are all translated fine linen. The word *byssus*, from Hebr. *batz*, has sometimes been supposed to indicate cotton; but as Herodotus uses the word *byssine sindon* to indicate the mummy-cloth, and as *sindon* is supposed to be derived from *Sindus* or *Indus*, it has been inferred that this was cotton; but microscopical observations in every case have shown, that linen alone was used for mummy-cloth (v. Bauer, Ure, and nob. Illustr. p. 85), notwithstanding that the contrary is stated by Rosselini.

But that cotton was known in Egypt at a very early period, we have the proofs, in Herodotus describing a coat of mail sent as a present by Amasis to the Samians, which was made of tree-wool: even in the present day, Indians wear cotton-padded coats, which are sword-proof. Nearchus, who visited India about a century later than Herodotus, and travelled in Egypt, has no one word to express the cotton dress of the Indians: he says that it is made of flax from trees (λινου του απο των δενδρεων), (Egypt. Antiq. ii. p. 125.) But Arrian, the author of the Periplus, uses a word evidently derived from the Sanscrit *karpasa*; Hindee, *kapas*. The Latin *Carbasus*, used for sails by Virgil and Cicero, fine clothes by Propertius, fine tent cloths by Pliny, pointed out to me by my learned colleague, the Rev. Professor Browne, seems also to be derived from this source. So, *Carpas*, employed in the book of Esther, i. 6, is evidently the same word, which Scheuzhzer, in his "Physica Sacra," conjectured was cloth of Asbestos or Amianthus;* but a

* The passage alluded to in Esther, is that of the description of the Court of the garden of the King's palace, where were white, green, and blue hangings, fastened with cords of fine linen and purple to silver rings and pillars of marble. It has been remarked, that cloth of amianthus could never have been got in sufficient quantities for these hangings; while, to Dr. Taylor's opinion of its being calico, it has been objected, that it seems insufficient to answer the purpose of an *awning*, from the thinness of its texture. To this it may be replied, that tents made of it, of several folds, withstand all weathers. Hanging curtains made

with

note to this article by the editor of Harris's Dictionary, fully explains the meaning—" *karpasus* occurs in the Periplus of Arrian, and is rendered by Dr. Vincent *fine muslin*. It is derived from the Sanscrit *karpasi;* from which probably the Hebrew word is also derived." "Similarity of name," Dr. Vincent has elsewhere said, " is a corroborating circumstance, when we are sure of our position; but till the position be ascertained, it is only a presumptive proof, and often fallacious."

Having indicated the several routes of ancient commerce, as well as the substances which it embraced, we may conclude the subject with a few words respecting the places whence these several articles were brought into Egypt and Palestine. The only ones specifically mentioned are, Ophir and Tharshish. Both of these, according to Heeren, indicate the rich countries of the south, such as the east coast of Africa, and Ceylon with the Peninsula of India, rather than any particular places; though the ships are described as returning every three years. This has been interpreted as meaning every third year; the voyage therefore may not have occupied so much as two years of time; and this is not more than would be necessary in the infancy, and during the practice, of coasting navigation; in addition to the time consumed in the dilatory modes of parting with the old, and taking in a new cargo, as well as that often required by the necessity of waiting for the monsoons.

with calico, usually in stripes of different colours, and padded with cotton, called *purdahs*, are employed throughout India, as a substitute for doors. They may be seen used for the very purposes mentioned in the text, in the court of the King of Delhi's palace, where on a paved mosaic terrace, rows of slender pillars, support a light roof, from which hang by rings immense padded and striped curtains, rolled up or removable at pleasure. These either increase light or ventilation, and form, in fact, a kind of moveable wall to the structure, which is used as one of the halls of audience, and was probably introduced by the Persian conquerors of India, and therefore explains the object of the colonnade in front of the palace in the ruins of Persepolis.

From the passages in which the above places are mentioned, we learn that "the King's (Solomon) ships went to Tharshish with the servants of Hiram: every three years once came the ships of Tharshish, bringing gold and silver, ivory, and apes and peacocks." (2 Chron. ix. 21.) In connexion with this may be adduced the passage of Ezekiel (xxvii. 12): "Tharshish was thy merchant by reason of the multitude of all kinds of riches; with silver, iron, tin and lead, they traded in thy fairs." From the mention of tin and lead as merchandize procured from Tharshish, it has been concluded that this must be Tartessus in Spain, though it is as probable that the name was subsequently given to this, when found to yield products previously obtained from the East; as no doubt some place in the West is intended (Jonah i. 4), for which Joppa is the port of embarkation. But that another, and therefore most likely the original Tharshish, was in the East, is rendered at least probable by its being mentioned with eastern ports, as in Ezek. xxxviii. 13: "Sheba and Dedan, and the merchants of Tharshish:" but of this there can, I conceive, be no doubt, when we find that the ships went to Tharshish from Eziongaber, in the eastern gulf of the Red Sea. As in 2 Chron. xix. 36: "And he, Jehosaphat, joined himself with him (Ahaziah, King of Israel), to make ships to go to Tharshish—and the ships were broken, that they were not able to go to Tharshish." That Ophir and Tharshish were in the same direction seems evident, from reference to the same occurrence, in 1 Kings, xxii. 48: "Jehosaphat made ships of Tharshish to go to Ophir for gold: but they went not; for the ships were broken at Eziongaber." From Ophir were obtained gold, algum or almug trees, and precious stones. Dr. A. Clarke adduces the Arabic version, as considering Ophir and Tharshish to refer to India; and my friend, Mr. C. Groves, has called my attention to Seba and Havilah, being considered by the

Targum, as referring to Sinde and Hinde; and Ophir being explained, as the place whence gold, and Havilah as that whence pearls were brought.

From these several products, especially ivory, apes, peacocks, and pearls, it is evident that only southern countries, whether Africa or India, could have been the object of these voyages. But cinnamon and cassia, nard, calamus, and onycha, having been shown to be peculiar Indian products, known to ancient commerce; there can, I conceive, be no doubt that the west coast of India, and probably also the island of Ceylon, were reached even in those early times. This is the more probable, as the voyages were commenced in the Red Sea, and occupied three years, or returned every third year.

The above details may appear to have little reference to Hindoo Medicine, or Materia Medica; but Hindoo Chronology has been justly doubted, and in consequence of claiming too much, their antiquity as an early educated and highly civilized nation has been entirely denied. It was incumbent therefore to show, on undoubted and extrinsic grounds, that they were well known to, and highly estimated by, ancient contemporary nations; that the valued natural products of their country were not more the objects of constant research than were the highly-prized specimens of their manufacturing skill.

Considering, therefore, these points as proved, we may be the less disinclined to consider their claims to literary and scientific originality; without at all giving credit to their own most extravagant dates, which may probably be most correctly considered, as only multiplications of astronomical periods. Since the testimony of those favourable to their claims, though best acquainted with their literature; might be received with doubt, as being opinions formed under the influence of a favourable bias: it will be preferable to adduce the admission of one, whose "mania for modernizing renders his testimony of the advanced knowledge of the Hindoos in astronomy, at so remote a period as the fifteenth century before Christ, the more valuable." My friend, Mr. Prinsep, moreover remarks in his Indian Chronological Tables, p. 78, "that there is great uncertainty and incongruity in many of Bentley's determinations of the dates of native princes and of books, from the prejudices he exhibits." This is evident, also, from his having chosen that for the classic age of Hindoo literature, (A.D. 1183, Heeren, vol. iii. p. 128,) which is known to history as the unsettled period of the Mahomedan invasion of India. Besides this, we have shown that the Arabs translated their works in the eighth, and that the Persians did so as early as the fifth century of our era. But "he (Bentley) is entitled to every confidence in his ingenious mode of calculating the period at which the various improvements in astronomy were introduced, and the *Siddhantas* written or revised; by the time when the positions of the planets, as assigned by their tables, accorded best with the more accurate results of European astronomy. From the minimum errors, and the precession of the equinoxes (first applied to such a purpose by Sir Isaac Newton), we have the following epochs substantially ascertained."

Invention of the Nacshatras or Hindu Lunar Mansions, B.C. 1425. Bentley.
The Solar Zodiac, formed by *Parasara* (under *Yudhistira*) B.C. 1180. do.
A Lunar Cycle, invented and precession discovered (Rama ?) B.C. 945. do.

"The situation of the equinoctial colure in the time of the astronomer Parasara, who flourished under Yudhistira, is fixed by Davis in 1391 B.C., by Sir Wm. Jones, Colebrooke, and Bentley, in 1180; which latter closely accords with the epoch of the *Cycle of Parasurama*, used in the Dakhan, and apparently unknown to these authors, B.C. 1176." (Prinsep. l.c. p. 78.)

The two Sanscrit epic poems, called *Ramayana* and *Mahabharat*, of the poets Valmiki and Vyasa, are believed by some to have been revised and corrected by the Poet Calidas, in the reign of Vikramaditiya, whose era commences B.C. 57 (Prinsep). The poems therefore were probably written some centuries before, but are supposed by Bentley to have been composed, the first only in A.D. 291, and the second in A.D. 600, though their much greater antiquity is proved by the sculptures in the temples of Elephanta, &c. (Heeren, iii. p. 277.) The Puranas are believed to have been composed as late as from the eighth to the tenth centuries of our era.

But the above two poems, according to Heeren, form the second, while the age of Vikramaditiya, makes the third era of Hindoo literature. The Vedas are far more ancient than all—sufficiently so to contain no notices of Buddhism, nor of the different Indian sects; the worship of Rama and Krishna having succeeded to that of the Elements and Planets (Colebrooke). The Vedas are thought by Sir William Jones to be next in antiquity to the five books of Moses. (Disc. ix.) This most probably is intended to apply only to the three first, the fourth being always considered less ancient than the others. It is of this, or the Atharva Veda (note, p. 56), that the Ayur Veda, or medical writings of highest antiquity and authority are collectively called, are considered to be a portion. The two most ancient authors, Charaka and Susruta, are made contemporaries of Rama and of the heroes of the time of fable (p. 57); while Aghastier, the translator into Tamul of Sanscrit medical literature, is named in the Ramayana, "the oldest work in the profane literature of the Hindoos," and therefore prior, we may conclude, to the Christian era. Sir W. Jones, in referring to this work, says, that the "Ayur Veda, supposed to be the work of a celestial physician, is almost entirely lost:" "but I have myself met with curious fragments of that primeval work; and in the Veda itself, I found, with astonishment, an entire Upanishad on the internal parts of the human body; with an enumeration of the nerves, veins, and arteries; a description of the heart, spleen, and liver, and various disquisitions on the formation and growth of the fœtus." (Jones, Disc. xi.) "Physic appears in these regions to have been cultivated from time immemorial," "as well as chemistry, on which we may hope to find useful disquisitions in Sanscrit, since the old Hindoos unquestionably applied themselves to that enchanting study." (Jones, Disc. x.)

Besides the discussion of medical subjects in these very ancient works, we may infer the antiquity of Medicine among the Hindoos, from the high estimation in which the profession has been always held there, as is evident from "one of the *fourteen Retnas*, or precious things, which their gods are believed to have produced by churning the ocean with the mountain, Mandura was a *learned physician*." (Jones, Disc. 2) That medical substances were equally prized, we learn from the Sanscrit account of the Deluge, given in the first Purana, evidently from older works or traditions, where, among other directions, we find, "Then shalt thou take all *medicinal herbs*, all the variety of seeds, and accompanied by seven saints, encircled by pairs of all brute animals, thou shalt enter the spacious ark, and continue in it secure from the flood, on one immense ocean, without light, except the radiance of thy holy companions." (Jones on Gods of India, &c.) "He (Satyvrata), still meditating on the commands of Bhagavat, saw the vessel advancing, and entered it with the chiefs of Brahmans, having carried into it the *medicinal creepers*," &c. (v. Jones, l. c.)

Considering therefore the high probability, if it be

thought short of positive proof, that the works in which the earliest medical writings of the Hindoos are contained, are very ancient; we can hardly deny to them the early cultivation of medicine; and this so early, as, from internal evidence, to be second, apparently to none with whom we are acquainted. This is further confirmed by the Arabs and Persians early translating their works; so also the Tamuls and Cingalese in the south; the Tibetans and Chinese in the East; and likewise from our finding, even in the earliest of the Greek writers, Indian drugs mentioned by corrupted Sanscrit names. We trace them at still earlier periods in Egypt, and find them alluded to even in the oldest chapters of the Bible.

It has been remarked, that improvements in medicine have usually kept pace with those in the other sciences and arts of life. Medicine is not likely, therefore, to have attained any great perfection in India, without some traces of corresponding literary and scientific eminence. Nor, indeed, does India form any exception to the general observation, for in the histories of the sciences, we find constant reference to the East as having originated, or at least cultivated, and made improvements in several. To investigate so extensive a subject, or attempt to do justice to even one of its subdivisions, would require not only time and space, but that which is still less at my command, namely, a thorough knowledge of the history and progress of the sciences in question in other parts of the world, as well as of the language and early literary and scientific acquirements of the Hindoos. But as this ignorance of Sanscrit has no doubt deprived me of the power of tracing many words and names of material substances to their original sources, so it has given my opinions the advantage of being in a great measure unbiassed; because it was not from an acquaintance with, or fondness for their literature, that I was led to infer its originality; but, from studying the translations in Persian and Latin of the works of the Arabs, I felt, from the nature of the information, that much of it must have been borrowed from the Indians; and this was confirmed by their reference by name to the Hindoo Charaka, (v. p. 37.)

In this investigation, we get little assistance from the Hindoos themselves, in consequence of their extravagant claims having deprived their chronology of credit, even on the most moderate computations. But their stationary nature affords a peculiar advantage in drawing inferences; for in the present day, we find them the same in manners and in customs as in the time of Alexander, though with the addition in those early ages of a high character for wisdom; from which, like the modern Greeks, they have certainly now degenerated. This very stationary nature, however, appears to me a result of their early civilization; for frequently conquered as they have been, and ruled over by ruder nations, they have usually made these in some measure conform to their own higher notions of civilization, instead of adopting, or being corrupted, by the coarser manners of their earlier conquerors.

That "India early acquired a high character for the wisdom of its philosophers," we are informed by history; whence we learn, that "it was visited by Pythagoras, Anaxarchus, Pyrrho, and others, who afterwards became eminent philosophers in Greece." (Brucker's Philosophy by Enfield.) From Pliny we learn, "Certe Pythagoras, Empedocles, Democritus, Plato, ad hanc discendam navigare, exsiliis verius quam peregrinationibus susceptis. (Plin. xxx. c. 2.) Thales, Crates, and Eudoxus, are others who are stated to have travelled in the East; but we are unable to ascertain how far these travels extended, and must therefore have recourse to other evidence, to perceive if there be sufficient similarity either in sentiment or science to prove the likelihood of an early communication between the Greeks and Hindoos. There is, in the first place, no doubt that the fame of Indian philosophers was sufficiently great and extended, 300 years before the Christian era, to induce the conqueror of Asia, and enlightened pupil of Aristotle, Alexander, to visit and hold intercourse with some of the Indian Gymnosophists.

From the researches of our celebrated countrymen, Jones Colebrooke, and Wilson, assisted by the labours of many German and French Orientalists, we can now obtain, by consulting a variety of works, as well as Transactions of Societies, a general idea of Hindoo science and literature, as treasured up in the ancient Sanscrit. To these sources, therefore, and the abstracts made from them, I have been indebted for the information which follows, and which I have incorporated, that the argument may be viewed in its integrity, instead of in isolated details.

The very perfection and "highly polished grammatical structure," of the language, with which so many others are connected, and from which, or from some very ancient common source, they must have been derived, prove the great attention paid by the Hindoos to literature. Works on grammar, lexicography, and metrics, form altogether one of the main branches of Sanscrit literature. (v. "The Hindoos," ascribed to the late Dr. Rosen.) The classified dictionary, containing 10,000 words, called *Amera Cosha*, has frequently been quoted.

The Vedas have been mentioned as the most ancient, and also as the most important of the Hindoo works; forming the basis of their religion, as well as the foundation of their social and political institutions. The four, called the Rig, Yajur, Sama, and Atharva Veda, have their present arrangements attributed to the sage Vyasa.

Each Veda consists of two parts, denominated the *Mantras*, or prayers, and the *Brahmanas*, or precepts. Indra, or the firmament, fire, the sun, moon, water, air, the spirits, the atmosphere, and the earth, are the objects most frequently addressed. The language of a considerable portion is an obsolete, and frequently very obscure dialect of Sanscrit. From a passage, stating the position of the solstitial points, which occurs in a sort of calendar appended to the Rig Veda, Mr. Colebrooke, to whom we are chiefly indebted for our knowledge of the Vedas, concludes that this calendar must have been regulated in the fourteenth century B.C.

The Puranas, eighteen in number, though comparatively modern, are next in importance to the Vedas: they have been described as legendary poems, similar in some respects to the Grecian theogonies. An abstract of the contents of several has been given by Professor Wilson, in the Journal of the Asiatic Society of Calcutta. Each Purana treats of five subjects: the creation of the universe; its destruction, and the renovation of worlds; the avataras, or manifestations of the supreme deity; the genealogy of gods and heroes; chronology, according to a fabulous system; and heroic history, containing the achievements of demigods and heroes.

The poetry of the Hindoos may be mentioned after these great works; and the two great epic poems, the Ramayana and Mahabharat, remarkable for their antiquity, consist respectively of 24,000 and 100,000 stanzas. They have other extensive poems, which have been classed under the heads of narrative, didactic, lyric, and apologue. Upon the invention of the latter, the Hindoos especially pride themselves. Of their dramatic literature, a very favourable opinion has been formed from Sir Wm. Jones's translation of Sakuntala, and more especially from Professor Wilson's Hindoo Theatre, containing translations of six

Sanscrit dramas. The Indian origin of the Fables of Pilpay has been already mentioned; but some even of the tales of the Arabian Nights' Entertainments have been traced to the voluminous Sanscrit collection of stories, called *Vrihatkat'ha.*

Of the Hindoo systems of philosophy, Sir Wm. Jones has said, "we now live among the professors of those philosophical tenets, which the Ionic and Attic writers illustrated with all the beauties of their melodious language. In retired scenes, in groves, and in seminaries of learning, we may perceive the Brahmans and the Sarmanes, mentioned by Clemens, disputing in the forms of logic, or discoursing on the vanity of human enjoyments, on the immortality of the soul, her emanation from the eternal mind, her debasement, wanderings, and final union with her source. The six philosophical schools, whose principles are explained in the Dersana Sastra, comprise all the metaphysics of the Old Academy, the Stoa, the Lyceum; nor is it possible to read the Vedanta, or the many fine compositions in illustration of it, without believing that Pythagoras and Plato derived their sublime theories from the same fountain with the sages of India." (3d Disc.) "The little treatise, in four chapters, ascribed to Vyasa, is the only philosophical Sastra, the original text of which I have had leisure to peruse with a Brahmin of the Vedanti school." The commentary of Sancara on the Vedanta, "not only elucidates every word of the text, but exhibits a perspicuous account of all other Indian schools, from that of Capila to those of the more modern heretics. It is not possible, indeed, to speak with too much applause of so excellent a work; and I am confident in asserting, that, until an accurate translation of it shall appear in some European language, the general history of philosophy must remain incomplete. (Jones. 11th Disc.) The author of "The Hindoos" has, from Mr. Colebrooke's Essays, briefly noticed the systems of philosophy which are considered orthodox by the Hindoos, because consistent with the theology of the Vedas; as the two *Mimansa* schools: others, incompatible with their sacred writings, are deemed by them heretical; such are the *Nyaya* and the *Vaiseshika* system: others, again, are partly heterodox, and partly conformable to the established Hindoo creed; such are the *Sankhya* and *Yoga*. "The *Nyaya*, of which Gotama is the acknowledged author, furnishes a philosophical arrangement, with strict rules of reasoning, not unaptly compared to the dialectic of the Aristotelian school." While Kanade, the reputed author of the *Vaiseshika*, maintained, like Democritus, the doctrine of Atoms. (The Hindoos. ii. p. 317-321.)

My friend, Sir Graves Haughton, in his exposition of the Vedanta philosophy, has stated with respect to their philosophy, that "the androgynous characteristic of male and female principles, which is at the bottom of all Hindoo metaphysical systems, as well as the tendency of the language to personification and realism, has given a bias to their philosophy, which could not be corrected even by the wonderful power and acuteness of their metaphysicians. But for the taint arising from these causes, the system contained in Manu would be almost perfect; and if its unfathomable antiquity be also considered, it must be allowed to be the most extraordinary effort ever made by the mind of man. It is the undoubted prototype of every subsequent system, of which we have any knowledge, whether we call them Hindoo, Chinese, Egyptian, Persian, Chaldæan, or European, which are all but distorted and mutilated copies of this one grand, simple, and original conception, already given in one line. 1. God;—2. Mind;—3. Consciousness;—4. Matras;—5. Elements." "*Matras* are the invisible types of the visible atoms which compose the five elements—Æther, Air, Fire, Water, and Earth."

Sir Wm. Jones thinks, that by means of the Puranas, we shall in time discover all the learning of the Egyptians, without decyphering their hieroglyphics, and states having no doubt, that their Osiris and Isis are the Iswara and Isi of the Hindoos. They mean, he conceives, the powers of Nature, considered as male and female; and that Isa, like the other goddesses, represents the active power of her lord; whose eight forms, under which he becomes visible to man, were thus enumerated by Calidasa near two thousand years ago. "*Water* was the first work of the Creator; and *Fire* receives the oblation of clarified butter, as the law ordains: the sacrifice is performed with solemnity; the *two lights* of Heaven distinguish time; the subtle *Ether*, which is the vehicle of sound, pervades the Universe; the *Earth* is the natural parent of all increase; and by *Air*, all things breathing are animated. May Isa, the *power* propitiously apparent in these eight forms, bless and sustain you." (Jones, on the Gods, &c.)

In addition to what has been above-mentioned respecting the syllogistic form of reasoning, as in use among the ancient Hindoos, we may adduce the "tradition which prevailed, according to the well-informed author of the Dabistan, in the Punjab, and in several Persian provinces; that 'among other Indian curiosities, which Callisthenes transmitted to his uncle, was a *technical system of logic*, which the Brahmans had communicated to the inquisitive Greek,' and which the Mahomedan writer supposes to have been the ground-work of the famous Aristotelean method." (Jones. 11th Disc.)

Hindoo law has been a subject necessarily paid much attention to, from the peculiar position of the English in India; and the translations and comments of Sir W. Jones,

Mr. Colebrooke, and Sir Graves Haughton, give us ample information on this subject. The books of law are numerous, and form an important branch of Sanscrit literature, consisting both of compilations and commentaries. Among these, the Institutes of Menu are the most distinguished, and considered to have been written as early as 880 B.C. (Heeren). Some of their works contain maxims or precepts put together into codes, which are attributed to ancient sages, as their original and inspired authors; others consist either of comments on these traditional tracts, or of systematic treatises, in which the several topics of Hindoo jurisprudence are discussed according to logical arrangement; and passages from the ancient law-givers are adduced, in support of the doctrines advanced. (Hindoos. ii. p. 311.)

If from their literature and philosophy we pass to the science of the Hindoos, we shall find equal reason to conclude, that it was not only in vividness of imagination and powers of philosophical abstraction that they excelled, but that the exact sciences were equally cultivated, and apparently with an original and successful result. The essays and translations which we have on the subject of Hindoo Mathematics, are from the pens of Messrs. Colebrooke, Reuben Barrow, Edward Strachey, Dr. Taylor, of the Madras, and the late Mr. John Tytler, of the Bengal Medical service. Also by M. Bailly in his Astron. Ind., and the celebrated Playfair in the Edinb. Phil. Trans.; who both support the high antiquity of Hindoo science. The results of these essays have been ably abridged by Professor Wallace in British India, (Vol. iii. p. 401.) and by others.

The Sanscrit writings from which a knowledge of Hindoo mathematics has been obtained, are different astronomical works, in which most of their mathematical treatises are contained. In the admirable article on Arithmetic by Mr.

Peacock, in the Encyclopedia Metropolitana, the history of this science has been treated in a manner to leave us nothing to wish for. There, the claims of the Hindoos to the discovery of the decimal numeration, are fully treated of; though some circumstances in the construction of the numerical language of Tibet, have induced him to suspect that it may have originated in that country. But knowing since the investigations of Csoma de Köros, how much the Tibetans have copied from Sanscrit literature in the seventh century, we require further evidence before we can ascribe to them the invention of so perfect and commodious a system of numeration. It is considered by the Hindoos to be of divine origin, "the invention of nine figures, with device of place being asciibed to the beneficent Creator of the Universe." (Colebrooke, ex Bhascara, &c.) "If the invention is to be determined by the known antiquity of possession, we must certainly refer it to Hindostan, as from the internal evidence of their numerical language, the Hindoos must have possessed a very perfect system of arithmetic from great antiquity." The Sanscrit names, moreover, of the ten numerals have been adopted with slight variations, not merely in all languages of the same class and origin, but likewise in many others, which are radically different from them. It is hardly necessary to notice the opinion of the Arabian origin of the notation by nine digits and zero, as their own testimony is decisive of the source whence they derived it. "The first Arabian who wrote upon algebra, and the Indian mode of computation, is stated, with the common consent of Arabic authors, to have been Mahommed ben Musa, the Khuwarezmite, who flourished about the end of the ninth century; an author who is celebrated as having made known to his countrymen other parts of Hindoo science." (Peacock. l.c. p. 413.)

The systems of astronomy referred to, contain treatises

on the subject of arithmetic (*Lilavati*), algebra (*Vija Ganita*), geometry, and mensuration, by the astronomers Bramagupta, Bhascara, and Aryabhatta. "The *Lilavati* treats of arithmetic, and contains not only the common rules of that science,—there reckoned, eight in number,—but the application of these rules to various questions on interest, barter, mixtures, combinations, permutations, the science of progressions, indeterminate problems, and, lastly, of the mensuration of surfaces and solids." "The rules are found to be exact, and nearly as simple as in the present state of analytical investigation. The numeral results are readily deduced; and if they be compared with the earliest specimens of Greek calculation, the advantages of the decimal notation are placed in a striking light." (Wallace.)

"It appears from the Hindoo treatises on algebra, that they understood well the arithmetic of surd roots; that they knew the general resolution of equations of the second degree, and had touched on those of higher denomination, resolving them in the simplest cases; that they had attained a general solution of indeterminate problems of the first degree, and a method of deriving a multitude of answers to problems in the second degree, when one solution was discovered by trials. This is as near an approach to a general solution, as was made, until the time of Lagrange. The Hindoos had also attempted equations of higher orders: they not only applied algebra both to astronomy and geometry, but conversely applied geometry to the demonstration of algebraic rules." Mr. Colebrooke has, by a variety of arguments, shown that the astronomer and algebraist, Aryabhatta (the oldest of those they consider their uninspired and merely human writers), wrote as far back as the fifth century of the Christian era, and probably at a much earlier period: he was therefore, even on this computation, almost as old as the Greek algebraist, Diophantus, who lived about the year 360. Mr. Colebrooke has further instituted a comparison between the Greek and Hindoo algebraists, and found reason to conclude that, in the whole science, the former are very far behind the latter. He says, the points in which the Hindoo algebra appears distinguished from the Greek are, besides a better and more convenient algorithm:

1st. "The management of equations of more than one unknown quantity.

2d. "The resolution of equations of a higher order, in which, if they achieved little, they had at least the merit of the attempt.

3d. "General methods for the resolutions of indeterminate problems of the first and second degrees, in which they went far indeed beyond Diophantus, and anticipated discoveries of modern algebraists.

4th. "The application of algebra to astronomical investigations and geometrical demonstrations, in which they also hit upon some matters which have been re-invented in modern times."

Having determined the inferiority of the algebra of Diophantus; the degrees of improvement by which it advanced to its perfection, in the time of Aryabhatta, becomes the next question—was it known long before, or was it then only discovered. "The late Professor Playfair was of opinion, that it was much older. He observes, that it is generally acknowledged that Diophantus cannot, himself, have been the inventor of all the rules and methods which he delivers; much less is Aryabhatta to be held the sole inventor of a system that was still more perfect than that of Diophantus. Indeed, before an author could think of embodying a treatise of algebra in the heart of a system of astronomy, and turning the researches of the one science to the purposes of the other, both must be in such a state of advancement, as the lapse of several ages, and many repeated efforts of invention, were required to produce."

The treatises on geometry are pronounced to be inferior in excellence to those on algebra; but they contain the celebrated proposition, that the square on the hypothenuse of a right-angled triangle, is equal to the squares on the sides containing the right angle; and others which form part of the system of modern geometry. Among these, that which discovers the area of a triangle when its three sides are known, is remarkable, as it does not appear to have been known to the ancient Greeks.

The division of the circle among the Hindoos, and their correspondence in this respect with the Greeks, is a subject which has attracted attention; and deservedly so, as it is purely conventional, having no dependence on the nature of the circle. Of this the circumference is divided by the ancient Hindoos into 360 equal parts, each of which was subdivided into sixty, and these into an equal number of smaller parts, similar to our present division into degrees, minutes, and seconds. The Hindoos, moreover, express the radius of a circle in parts of the circumference, and have but one measure (the minute of a degree) for both. Of these, the circumference is said to contain 21,600, and the radius 3438, which is pronounced by mathematicians as great a degree of accuracy as can be obtained; without taking in smaller divisions than minutes, as it is true to the nearest minute; and this is all the exactness aimed at in their trigonometrical tables. The Bramins, however, knew to greater exactness the ratio of the diameter to the circumference, as they supposed it to be as 1 to 3.1416.

"The tables employed in their trigonometrical calculations are two,—one of sines, and the other of versed sines: the sine of an arc they call *cramajya* or *jyapinda*, and the versed sine *utcramajya*. These terms seem to be derived from the word *jya*, which signifies the chord of an arc, from which the name of the radius, or sine of 90°, *viz*. *trijya*, is also taken. This regularity in their trigonometrical language, is not unworthy of remark; but what is of more consequence to be observed is the use of sines, as it was unknown to the Greeks, who calculated by the help of the chords, and this forms a striking difference between theirs and the Indian trigonometry." The table of sines exhibits them to every twenty-fourth part of the quadrant; the table of versed sines does the same: in each, the sine, or versed sine, is expressed in minutes of the circumference, neglecting fractions. Thus, the sine of 3° 45′ is 225; the sine of 7° 30′ is 449; and so on. The rule for the computation of the sines is curious; it indicates a method of computing a table by means of their second differences,—a considerable refinement in calculation, and first practised by the English mathematician Briggs." (Wallace.)

The *Surya Siddhanta*, continues the author of the abridged essay on Hindoo Mathematics in British India, ii. p. 463, does not give the demonstration of the truth of the rule; but the commentary gives direct geometrical means for their calculation. In the progress of science, the invention of trigonometry is a step of great importance, and of considerable difficulty. He who first formed the idea of exhibiting, in arithmetical tables, the ratio of the sides and angles of all possible triangles, must have been a man of profound thought, and of extensive knowledge. However ancient, therefore, any book may be, in which we meet with a system of trigonometry, we may be assured that it was not written in the infancy of the science. We may therefore conclude, that geometry must have been known in India long before the writing of the *Surya Siddhanta*. Professor Playfair, speaking of the Indian rule for computing sines, which is certainly very ingenious, says, "It has the appearance, like many other things in the science of those eastern nations, of being drawn up by one who was more deeply versed in the subject than may be at first imagined, and who knew much more than he thought it necessary to communicate. It is probably a compendium formed by some ancient adept in geometry for the use of others, who were merely practical calculators."

Though the majority of writers allow the Hindoos credit for the originality and advanced state of their mathematics, it is very different with their astronomy, which, though equally supported by great names, such as those of Bailly and Playfair, and acquiesced in by Sir David Brewster, has been objected to as being neither ancient nor original; their astronomical books on the subject being conceived to be modern compilations, to which old names have been attached: the matter having been borrowed from the Greeks and Arabians. But equal fairness does not appear to me to be observed in the statement of the argument: for, allowing full force to the ingenuity and truth of the mode of reasoning, and induction from internal evidence, of the principal Hindoo astronomical works, as the *Brahma*, *Surya*, and *Arya Siddhantas* having been composed respectively in the years 538, 1068, and 1322, of the Christian era; yet the very same author proves by the same mode of induction, that the astronomer Parasara lived as early as 1180 B.C. The Hindoos must have paid attention to astronomy at even earlier periods, for Mr. Bentley also admits, that the Nacshatras, or Hindoo lunar mansions, were determined as early as 1425 B.C.; the solar zodiac not till 1180 B.C. by the above-named Parasara; and the lunar cycle in 945 B.C.

Sir David Brewster (Edinb. Encycl. Astronomy, p. 585), in introducing this subject, says, "The astronomical tables of the Indians are in our hands, and, with evidence almost as irresistible as that which attends the principles of the science, we can trace the remoteness of their origin, and survey the advancement of the human mind in the earliest ages of the world." He then mentions the three sets of tables, those of Siam, of Narsapour, of Chrishna-bouram, as well as the fourth set brought by M. Gentil from Tirvalore, after being instructed by the Brahmans in their methods of calculation. The celebrated Bailly, in his "Traité de l'Astronomie Indienne et Orientale," found that the epoch of the Tirvalore tables coincides with the year 3102 B.C. "These high pretensions to antiquity, have been defended by Professor Playfair with an acuteness of reasoning, and a clearness of illustration, peculiar to that eloquent writer." "La Place has endeavoured to prove, though not with his usual success, that the epoch of 3102 was invented for the purpose of giving a common origin in the zodiac to all the motions of the heavenly bodies, and that the tables have either been constructed or corrected in modern times; but he at the same time allows, that the remarkable accuracy of the mean motions assumed in their construction could have arisen only from very ancient observations." (Brewster. l.c.) Without supposing that there could have been any great attention paid to astronomy at this early period, it is singular "that we learn from Persian works, that there were formerly four bright stars, which pointed out the four cardinal points of the heavens; and it is a very remarkable coincidence, in which chance could have no share, that, about 3000 years before the Christian era, Aldebaran and Antares were situated exactly in the two equinoctial points, while Regulus and the Southern Fish were placed in the two solstices." (Brewster. l.c. p. 584.)

As a trigonometry was necessary for the settlement of

many important points in astronomy, so we have it incorporated in their works on this science, and acknowledged even by those adverse to the Hindoo claims, that in many points it is original, and in all highly curious. The circle, we have seen, was divided, for trigonometrical purposes, into 360 degrees, and each of these into sixty minutes; so the Hindoos divided time in a similar manner, that is, the year into six seasons, each of these consisting of 60 *dinas* (1 dina = 1 day and night); each dina = 60 dandas (1 danda = 24 minutes English); each danda = 60 palas (1 pala = 24 seconds); each pala = 60 vipalas (1 vipala = 0. 4 seconds); and so on for five more subdivisions for astronomical purposes. But the *daṇda* is also considered equal to sixty vicalas, each of which is equal to six respirations. From this coincidence in the division of the circle and of time, it has been supposed that the circle was divided into 360°, in consequence of the most ancient Hindoos supposing it to be the number of days in the year: this would even appear to be confirmed by their division of the year into six seasons of sixty dinas each = 360 days. But the number seems rather to have been adopted from the convenience of the sexagesimal division in calculations, as we learn that their tables "are founded on the supposition that the tropical year is $365^{d}\ 5^{h}\ 30'\ 40''$, a determination which differs only $1'\ 33''$ from that which is employed in the new solar tables of Delambre. (Brewster.)

Hindoo astronomy has been said to be confined to the calculation of certain changes in the heavens, particularly eclipses of the sun and moon, the places of the planets, with the rules and tables by which these calculations must be performed. They early distinguished the zodiac from the rest of the celestial sphere, and divided it into twenty-seven (Jones,) or twenty-eight (Colebrooke,) portions, which they call *nacshatras*, or asterisms, marking the moon's path in the heavens. The names of the Indian months are taken from twelve of these lunar mansions, or constellations of the solar zodiac, and this has been particularly remarked upon by the illustrious Humboldt. Time was besides divided into periods of seven days, "the most ancient monument of astronomical knowledge" (La Place); which has been supposed to have been formed from being nearly a fourth of twenty-seven days and seven hours, the time of a complete revolution of the moon through the zodiac; or perhaps from bearing the same proportion to twenty-nine and a-half days, the time of her passing through all her phases; or as probably from the tradition of the time in which the world was created. But it is remarkable that the days of the Hindoo week are, like those of the Egyptian and our own, named after the seven heavenly bodies, but with this difference, that Friday is the first day of their week. Thus, to take Wednesday as an example, which is named from *Woden* of the Scandinavians, who is the *Wud* and *Bud* of the Pagan Arabs, *Buddha* of the Hindoos, *Buddas* and *Sarmanes* of the Greeks, probably from the Sanscrit *Maha-sramana;* in which language he is also called *Mayà-devi-suta*, or child of Maya, the "Mercurius Mayæ filius" of Horace. The planet Mercury is in Sanscrit called *Bouta*, and the day of Mercury, *Boota varam*, or *Boodh-var.;* Hindee, *Boodh;* "Mercurii dies," or Wednesday, (v. Prinsep. l.c. 14 and 87.) Whatever else may be denied, this at least must be admitted, that the concurrence of the Hindoos and Egyptians, in similarly naming the days of the week, must have had a common origin; and that both were anterior to the Greeks.

"Besides their lunar zodiac, the Hindoos had another divided into twelve signs of 30° each. This was purely mathematical, and served for the purposes of calculation.

The divisions of this, their solar zodiac, were distinguished by names and emblems; and what is truly remarkable, they are the same as those which are connected with the signs of our own zodiac." It has been supposed that the Hindoos borrowed this from the Arabs; but Mr. Colebrooke has observed, "we know that the Hindoos have preserved the memory of a former situation of the colures compared to constellations, which make divisions of the zodiac in their astronomy; but no similar trace remains of the use of the lunar mansions, as divisions of the zodiac, among the Arabs in so very remote times."

The above perfect identity of the Hindoo zodiac with ours, will appear from the names of their signs. *Mesha*, the ram; *Vrisha*, the bull; *Milhuna*, the pair; *Carcata*, the crab; *Sinha*, the lion; *Canga*, the virgin; *Tula*, the balance; *Vrishahica*, the scorpion; *Dhanus*, the bow; *Macaru*, the sea-monster; *Cumbha*, the ewer; *Mina*, the fish. The zodiac itself they call *sodi-mandalam*. The coincidences here must have had a common source: not only do the signs nearly correspond with those of the Egyptian zodiac of the temple of Denderah, but also with those known to the Chaldeans.

The chief object of ancient astronomy for many ages was the proper settlement of time; this the Hindoos attained very successfully and without the assistance of other nations; though the Chinese, who claim great antiquity of observation, required that of the Arabs in A.D. 1290, and of the Jesuits in 1664. "There are a great variety of eras in use in different parts of India, but all may be classified under four general heads, according to the mode of expressing, or of subdividing the year; namely, first, those which are founded on the sidereal division of the months; secondly, those which follow the intricate and peculiar luni-solar computations; thirdly, those reckoned by cycles, and in which the years are distinguished by names, a system which spread from India into Tibet, and was long before used in China and Japan; and, fourthly, those derived essentially from the Muhammedan era," Prinsep. l.c. p. 17; from Col. Warren's *Kala Sankalita*, which, he says, "should be in the hands of every one desirous of obtaining a thorough knowledge of the subject."

The Hindoo solar year, as it is improperly called, is strictly sidereal. The solar zodiac was formed from the lunar one, about the year 1180 B.C., according to Bentley; the names of the months being taken from those of the lunar mansions, in which the moon happened to be full, in the year of its invention. The adoption of the fixed sidereal zodiac of twelve signs is ascribed by the same author to about A.D. 538, to which time the use of the solar zodiac lasted. This subject it is impossible to enter into: it may suffice to remark, that "the effect, on *civil reckoning*, is to produce differences in the relative lengths of the months, of one or even two days more, or one day less, and to bring about a bissextile year of 366 days, as nearly as possible once in four years." (Prinsep.)

"The circumstances of the Indian luni-solar year differ from every other mode of dividing and recording time, that has been employed in ancient or modern times. Some similarity had been observed in the secular omission of a month in the Chaldean system, and at a particular period the common intercalations concurred with those of the lunar cycle of Meton, which led the learned to imagine them derived from the same source; but Col. Warren has proved, from a minute analysis of the Hindoo *Chandra Mana*, that it has no further similitude to other systems than its dependence on the moon's motions must naturally indicate."

Of years numbered by cycles, that called the era of

Parasurama derives its name from a prince, who is supposed to have reigned 1176 B.C., the epoch being 7th August, 3537 Jul. Per., or 1925 Kal-yug. This era is reckoned in cycles of 1000 years. The commencement of the 977th year of the 3d cycle concurs with the 14th Sept. A.D. 1800.

The cycle of Jupiter is supposed by many to be one of the most ancient modes of reckoning time, not only in India, but in Asia generally: in the former, it is comparatively of modern introduction (A.D. 965-6,) v. Prinsep. l.c. p. 29; but it has been known in China from time immemorial, where it partakes of the same peculiarity as on the continent of India, of having separate names for each year of the cycle.

From the difficulty of ascertaining the extent to which the more modern of the Hindoo astronomers were indebted to their more ancient predecessors, it is impossible at present to determine how many of the doctrines which their works contain are entirely original. This will be easier, when we possess more translations, and are able to trace opinions to earlier sources, even from hints in works on other subjects. In the mean time it may be stated that the Hindoos were early acquainted with the spherical figure of the earth, and that they conceived it to be self-balanced in space. And though, like the Greeks, they had their epicycles and eccentrics, and there are coincidences in their system of calculating the inequalities of the sun, moon, and planets, they yet seem to have been ignorant of the modifications made in those hypotheses by Ptolemy. They knew that the moon revolves once a month on her axis; and that she was distant from the earth 220,184 geographical miles, which is 20,000 less than has been determined by European astronomers. To find the latitude of a place, they observed the length of the shadow of a perpendicular gnomon, when the sun is in the equator; and computed by their geometry the angle which the gnomon makes with the line drawn from its top to the extremity of the shadow. The longitude is directed to be found by observations of lunar eclipses, calculated for the meridian of Lanca, which passes through Oujein, one of their most ancient cities. The obliquity of the ecliptic they considered equal to 24° (the Chinese also state it to be 24°, but from their dividing the circle into 365¼°, this is only equal to 23° 39′.) The precession of the equinoxes they reckoned equal to fifty-four seconds in a year, but it is actually four seconds less than they supposed.

Though it is difficult to prove, whether or not, the Indians were indebted to the Greeks for any of their principal determinations, Mr. Davis and Delambre, both opposed to the great antiquity of the Hindoo astronomy, think their methods of calculation essentially different from the Grecian, and that those for eclipses, though tedious, are curious, and bear the appearance of originality. One of the most striking instances of this, is the method given in the tables of Chrisnabouram, for finding the time of the sun's continuance above the horizon, or what is called the diurnal arc for any given day. From the rule given not being rigorously true, and the differences between the supposition of the Brahmins and the exact formula, being very appreciable in high, but inconsiderable in tropical latitudes; it is evident that the rule which they adopt must have had its origin in a tropical country; and in all probability in the Indian Peninsula where it is found. (Playfair.)

Among the objections made to Hindoo astronomy, there is one which I think susceptible of explanation; and that is, their want of instruments, or modes of making observations. To this it may be replied, that in the Vishnu Dhermotter, it is directed that the planets be observed with an instrument: and in their method for determining the length of the solar year, the amplitudes, or rather their differences, are directed to be determined by marking the sun's position at rising, on a horizontal circle of considerable magnitude. Besides which, the astronomical buildings at Benares, Delhi, and Jyepoor, though all probably only a few centuries old, indicate the purposes for which they were required; and these purposes we have seen are not of very recent date among the Hindoos. The present buildings therefore may be of modern origin, but we cannot expect them to be ancient in a country, where, from the perishable nature of the materials employed in architecture, cities have succeeded cities, leaving scarcely any traces of their sites. These structures may, however, and most probably have, only succeeded others of a similar kind, but of much older date. That of Benares has been described by Sir R. Baker in the Philosophical Transactions for 1775; those of Jyepore and Delhi I have not seen described, but at the latter place, the large and lofty circular roofless building, or rather wall, pierced with horizontal rows of openings like windows, would seem as if intended to be employed for the purposes of a horizontal circle.

Mr. J. Bentley, in his papers in the Asiatic Researches, vols. vi. and viii., has inferred from the minimum errors in the Surya Siddhanta, that it was composed about A.D. 1067, and this is confirmed by other circumstances (v. Prinsep. Tables, p. 29): he also concludes that Varaha-mihira was the author of this work. But by reasoning entirely analogous to that with respect to the Surya Siddhanta, he was led to conclude that the system of astronomy, composed by Brahma-gupta, may be referred to A.D. 536; and this date nearly agrees with that assigned to the Brahma-Siddhanta by the Hindoos themselves. Now Mr. Colebrooke has observed, that Brahma-gupta, in a work of acknowledged authenticity, quotes by name Varaha, who flourished in A.D. 499 according to other authorities, (v. Prinsep. l.c. p. 79.) "Indeed it appears that Brahma-gupta was preceded by other astronomers, and particularly by one named Aryabhatta, deserving of notice here, as having advocated the doctrine of the earth's diurnal revolution on its axis, and who fixed the length of the sidereal year at 365 days 6 hours 12′ and 30″. These doctrines of Aryabhatta (called *Arjebahar* by the Arabs) render it a very interesting point to determine his age, that we may ascertain whether he borrowed this philosophical idea from the sages of Greece, or whether Pythagoras, who was undoubtedly well versed in the learning of the East, borrowed it himself from the Indians. But at present we have not sufficient data to decide this question, which is worthy of all the attention of Sanscrit scholars." v. from Asiat. Res. xii. p. 221 and 227; History of Astronomy. L. U. K. p. 11 and 12; where the arguments for and the objections against the antiquity of Indian astronomy are fairly adduced.

Sir W. Jones has affirmed it as improbable, that the Brahmins should have borrowed from other nations, especially the Greeks, whom they despised in particular; quoting a proverb, which he says they have, that no base creature can be lower than a Yavan; which is their term for an Ionian or Greek. But in his third Discourse, he states that "the philosopher whose works are said to include a system of the universe, founded on the principle of attraction and the central position of the sun, is named Yavan Acharya, because he had travelled, we are told, into Ionia. If this be true, he might have been one of those who conversed with Pythagoras. This at least is undeniable, that a work on astronomy in Sanscrit, bears the title of Yavan Jatica, which may signify the Ionic sect." This work I do not find elsewhere mentioned, but Mr. Colebrooke quotes a very curious passage from Varaha-mihira, where he says, that "the Yavans are barbarians; but this science is well established among them, and they are revered like holy sages." (As. Res. xii. p. 245.) This no doubt proves, what however does not require proof, that the Hindoos were acquainted with the Greeks. We know, indeed, that they made use of some of their inventions, as that of coinage (v. p. 72), prior even to the above age of Varaha-mihira. But the fact also proves that the Hindoos must themselves have previously paid attention to astronomy, to be able to appreciate the advances made by the Greeks.

If this admission by Hindoo astronomers of the time of Varaha, of an acquaintance with the cultivation of astronomy by the Greeks, be thought valuable, how much more so, for the purpose of ascertaining priority of scientific cultivation, is the constant reference, by the earliest Grecian writers, to the East, as the source of literature and of science, as well as the object of their travels in pursuit of knowledge, at much earlier periods than those of Varaha: the value of whose testimony, however, must necessarily be diminished, if his antiquity be reduced.

Before quitting the subject, it is proper to allude to the similarity which exists in the ancient astronomy of many Eastern nations. For though we may satisfy some minds by saying, that the Hindoos borrowed from the Arabs, these from the Greeks,—and therefore the coincidences between the first and the last; this will not account for the many points of agreement which exist between the Chinese and the Hindoos, as also between these and the Egyptians. Neither will it explain how the latter, as well as the Chaldeans, are reported as having been able to predict eclipses; and that methods for doing so, essentially different from the Grecian, exist in the oldest of the Hindoo astronomical works.

If the points of coincidence, from the prevalence of similar doctrines among the Greeks and Hindoos, appear remarkable, the absence among both, of the same sciences, is not less so. Thus, though the Hindoos, like the Egyptians, must have been acquainted with many mechanical powers, they do not seem to have cultivated mechanics as a science; nor hydrostatics, though, like the Chinese, they employed clepsydræ for the measurement of time. Neither though they knew that air was the vehicle of sound, do they seem to have studied its other properties; nor, though they had mirrors, and acquainted as they were with the fact of the angle of incidence being equal to the angle of reflection, do they seem to have made any further advance in optics. But neither was any great progress made in these sciences among the Greeks until later ages, as those of Archimedes and Ptolemy.* If the Hindoos, therefore, borrowed from the Greeks, they must have done so previous to these times, of 200 B.C. and 150 A.D. In the same way we have inferred, that if they borrowed medicine, they must have done so before the time of Galen; and therefore about the period when the peripatetic sages of Greece themselves

* This may be seen by consulting the valuable work of Mr. Whewell, on the History of the Inductive Sciences, which having appeared since the Lecture, of which this is a continuation, was delivered, and the greater portion of the foregoing pages printed, I have not been able to make the use of that I could have wished. I am pleased to find that, though inclined to the opinion of the early efforts in physical speculations, and their philosophy on such subjects, being the native growth of the Greek mind, and owing " nothing to the supposed lore of Egypt and the East; an opinion which has been adopted with regard to the Greek philosophy in general by the most competent judges, on a full survey of the evidence,"—he yet makes an exception, "perhaps of the Indians, as the only one of the African or Asiatic nations, who ever felt the importunate curiosity with regard to the definite application of the idea of cause and effect to visible phœnomena." p. 32. But that the Greeks received their first impulse in some of these studies from without, is shown in a subsequent page, (161,) where a quotation is made from Plato; where, after speaking of the Egyptians and Syrians as the original cultivators of astronomical studies, he adds, " Whatever we Greeks receive from the barbarians, we improve and perfect."

travelled in quest of knowledge throughout eastern regions. Hence, if we deny originality to the Hindoos, we cannot but allow them antiquity of application to scientific pursuits.

The sciences more particularly cultivated by the Hindoos, we have already noticed, and proved or at least shown the extreme probability, of the Arabs having been indebted to them for their first knowledge of Chemistry, as well as of some portion of their Medicine. The Hindoo Materia Medica being extensive, and comprising substances from the animal, vegetable, and mineral kingdoms, would indicate their having turned their attention, at least, to these departments of nature. But from the imperfect knowledge we possess of their books, it is impossible to say whether they contain any attempts at a scientific classification; or if they ever advanced from the observation of facts to generalisations of principles. That their arrangements sometimes proceeded beyond a merely alphabetical one, we see even in their dictionary, the *Amera Cosha*, which is arranged in a great measure according to subjects. The mineral kingdom they must necessarily have obtained some knowledge of, from their cultivation of chemistry. The vegetable articles of the Materia Medica, we have already seen, are grouped according to a system, adopted in even our latest and best books, as those of Martius and Guibourt; that is, according to the part of the plant employed, or the nature of the product collected (v. p. 54). From the familiarity with which Indian gardeners talk of male and female plants, it would appear that the Hindoos had obtained some knowledge of the sexes of plants. So also the rules which are given for the collection of medicines, and the properties of plants as connected with the climate and soil in which they grow; indicate that they generalised as well as observed. For not only is the kind of climate and soil mentioned, but also the characteristics of the inhabitants, their prevailing diseases, with the peculiarities of the vegetation, and the nature of the products it affords. The soil and climate where salutary or unwholesome plants grow, or those abounding in juices, or such as yield resins or oil, are likewise indicated; so the particular seasons are specified, when the different parts of officinal plants should be collected. Whether their knowledge of animals extended beyond mere acquaintance with their external forms, and the names by which they were known, I have no means of determining: but it is remarkable that the incarnations of their god Vishnu, should be in conformity to the modern views respecting the gradation of animal forms, as displayed in ascending from the less to the more highly developed; so the incarnations proceed from the fish to the tortoise, thence to the pachydermatous boar, the carnivorous lion, dwarf, Rama, &c.

From their Sciences we may proceed to the Fine Arts. Of these, the early cultivation of Poetry among the Hindoos has been already noticed; as well as their earliest Architecture for its resemblance to the Egyptian. Their later and more ornate style, is rich, beautiful, and peculiar; it may be seen in some still very ancient temples, and is represented in a few works, as Prinsep's Views of Benares, and the Treatise on Hindoo Architecture, by Ram Raz. Sculpture also early attracted the attention of the Hindoos; but though they never attained any great eminence in this department, their older are more perfect than their modern performances; for even in the ancient, nearly sea-covered, city of Mahabalipuram, some of the sculptures are stated by Bishop Heber to be very beautifully executed. Their Painting, known of course only in its modern state, does not proceed beyond indifferent likenesses, and faithfully copying what is put before them. But Music must be very ancient among the Hindoos, as it is treated of in one of the Upavedas, with Medicine, Warfare, and Mechanics. The Hindoos relate many marvellous stories respecting the effects of their ancient music, while they confess its decline in modern times. Sir Wm. Jones believed "that the Hindoo system of music has been formed on truer principles than our own; all the skill of the native composers is directed to the great object of their art, the natural expression of strong passions, to which indeed melody is often sacrificed; though some of their tunes are pleasing even to a European ear. Nearly the same may be truly asserted of the Arabian or Persian system; and by a correct explanation of the best books on that subject, much of the old Greek theory may probably be recovered." (Jones. 2d Disc.)

From this slight view of the Fine, the transition is easy to the Useful Arts of India; but this is a subject, which even more than the other has been neglected by Orientalists, though the results of inquiry might not only be practically useful, but would be extremely interesting. As many probably remain unchanged, we might be enabled to explain various processes of ancient times, by comparing old descriptions with modern practice; and also obtain some ideas respecting their attainments in science, from the applications made of it to practice. In previous pages (p. 98, 130, and 137), the success of the Hindoos in many mechanical and chemical arts has been mentioned. That commerce early attracted their attention, we have the assurance in the first of their sacred law tracts, (supposed to have been revealed by Menu, it is thought about 800 or 900 years before the Christian era), containing "a curious passage on the legal interest of money, and the limited rate of it in different cases, with an exception in regard to adventures at sea; an exception which the sense of mankind approves, and which commerce absolutely requires; though it was not before the reign of Charles I., that our jurisprudence fully admitted it in respect to maritime contracts." (Jones, 3d Disc.)

Among the useful arts, Agriculture, Weaving, Embroidering, Dyeing, Calico-printing, Working in Metals, and Pottery, the manufactory of Sugar and Indigo, were probably most conspicuous. That other useful arts have long been very numerous among the Hindoos is evident, for Sir Wm. Jones says, "that Europeans enumerate more than two hundred and fifty mechanical arts, by which the productions of nature may be variously prepared for the convenience and ornament of life; and though the Silpi Sastra (or Sanscrit Collection of Treatises on Arts and Manufactures,) reduces them to sixty-four, yet Abul Fazl had been assured that the Hindoos reckoned three hundred arts and sciences: now their sciences being comparatively few, we may conclude that they anciently practised at least as many useful arts as ourselves." (Jones, 10th Disc.) With respect to their skill in many of these arts, we may adduce the unexceptionable evidence of the late excellent, widely and universally esteemed Bishop Heber. "To say that the Hindoos or Musulmans are deficient in any essential feature of a civilized people, is an assertion which I can scarcely suppose to be made by any who have lived with them. Their manners are at least as pleasing and courteous, as those of the corresponding stations of life among ourselves; their houses are larger, and, according to their wants and climate, to the full as convenient as ours; their architecture is at least as elegant. Nor is it true, that in the mechanic arts they are inferior to the general run of European nations. Where they fall short of us (which is chiefly in agricultural implements, and the mechanics of common life), they are not, so far as I have understood of Italy and the south of France, surpassed in any great degree by the people of those countries."

Before concluding this view of the progress made by the ancient Hindoos in science and the arts, it would be extremely interesting to compare, what is contained in Sanscrit books on these several subjects, with what was known to the Greeks at the earliest period of their philosophical and scientific history. By this means we might in some measure ascertain the times, at which the communication chiefly occurred between the sages of the West, and those of the East; as undoubtedly the numerous coincidences which exist between the two cannot be accidental. Since the progress of scientific discoveries in those ages, must necessarily have been even more gradual than it has been since; we might consider them a series of epochs; which, correctly registered as they are among the Greeks, would give us dates for ascertaining when the Hindoos borrowed from them, by the absence in Sanscrit works of the later advances of science in the West. But if the preponderance of evidence should induce us to determine that the course of discovery, like the transit of tropical products, was from south to north, and from east to west: we might, in like manner, ascertain the times when the Hindoo discoveries (as, that of decimal notation) were made. Since these when less ancient would be unknown to the earlier Greeks, who appear to have been acquainted, with whatever constituted the early stock of Oriental knowledge, whencesoever derived.

I regret that this task has not been undertaken by some one competent to the task, though it may be difficult to find many such; for it requires not only a knowledge of the language in which much of the information is still clothed; but also of the classical works in which alone the scientific discoveries of the ancients are detailed. To this must be added an acquaintance with the several sciences, their history and principles; because hints or expressions of a general nature, which are perfectly intelligible to those acquainted with a science, are usually passed without observation by those, who look at an author only in a literary point of view. It is not because I have myself been addicted to the study of natural history, that I consider a knowledge of it equally requisite, for investigating this subject and determining the question of priority. But because only those, acquainted with the almost immutable laws, which control the distribution of vegetable and animal forms, perceive and feel the full force of the inferences to be deduced; from the presence of the products of plants in particular places, which could not be those of their growth. A Naturalist would at the same time, be more likely to discover, from the peculiarities of animal and vegetable physiology; whether opinions were not rather formed in other climates, than in those in which they are promulgated.

In prosecuting this subject, some assistance will, eventually, no doubt, be afforded by the Hindoos, who are now so zealously employed in studying the English language and European science. Some of them will probably conjoin with these a study of their own ancient language, and trace in it some of the earliest indications of sciences, which have been fully developed only in the countries of the West. Much aid will also be obtained from the prosecution of the translations which are now making from the Sanscrit, into Latin and several European languages. But the assistance here is less than might be expected, from the translations as yet chiefly consisting of works of a literary nature. But even these, when read by those versed in the several sciences, will often indicate the knowledge which had been attained on scientific subjects in the countries where they were written; and will, therefore, be available for the above purpose, until more of the treatises on the sciences, and some of those on the arts, are translated.

In entering upon this investigation, it is unnecessary to prove, that there was communication between the Hindoos and Greeks, because this we have seen, was both direct, and by means as well of Egypt as of Persia. But it cannot fail to strike one as remarkable, that, accustomed as the Greeks were to call all other nations, barbarians, they yet speak with respect of the Gymnosophists, or naked sages of India, called "Sapientes Indi" by Pliny. Also that we so constantly read in the early history of Greece, of Grecian sages travelling in Eastern regions, not for the purposes of communicating, but for acquiring information. We also learn, that many, on their return, established schools of instruction, from which emanated many important discoveries. These are not more remarkable for their value, than for precisely coinciding with those we now find recorded in Sanscrit works. At the same time, we hear nothing of the sages of the East visiting the certainly younger civilization of the West; and yet if we suppose them enlightened enough to borrow, we might expect that they had zeal enough to travel, in quest of the information, which in any case they evidently knew how to appreciate.

The first point worthy of observation, is the similarity of the subjects, upon which some of the earliest of the ancient Greeks wrote, and those which we now find contained in Sanscrit books. The coincidence between the philosophical systems of the Hindoos, and those of Plato and Pythagoras, who both travelled in the East, has been already mentioned. So also the immense mass of information collected by Theophrastus, and his general observations respecting Plants, and their distribution in different countries and soils, resemble in some measure the

Hindoo observations on similar subjects, and their attention to such subjects may, perhaps, account for the knowledge by the Greeks of Indian plants. In like manner, some of the views of Aristotle on the generation of animals, more especially that denominated equivocal, do not seem to differ from such as are found among the Hindoos. The early poet and physician Nicander wrote on poisons and their antidotes; so we have seen that this was one of the subjects early treated of by the Hindoos; and even that the Hindoo Manka translated a treatise on poisons from Sanscrit into Persian at the Court of Harun-al-Rashid. (v. p. 64.)

For these reasons, the several subjects on which Democritus wrote, have been mentioned at p. 115. That he travelled in southern regions, we have the proof in his having described the sensitive plant—his coincidence in opinion with the Hindoo Kanade respecting atoms, has already been stated—and it is curious that he should be cited as one of the earliest writers on chemistry (v. Enc. Metrop. Chemistry, p. 590), when it was not suspected that chemistry had ever been cultivated in the East, in the days when he travelled. Thus, likewise Eudoxus, who lived 370 years before the Christian era, and is said to have studied thirteen years in Egypt, is stated by Seneca to have introduced from thence into Greece, the theory of the five planets. "Eudoxus quinque syderum cursus in Græciam ab Ægypto transtulit." (Quæst. Nat. vii. 3.) He composed also a description of the sphere, which is supposed to have been copied from one long anterior to his own time, in consequence of his asserting that there is a certain star in the celestial sphere, corresponding to the pole of the equator. "Now this could not have been the polar star of our times, which was then, owing to the precession of the equinoxes, far from the pole; and upon examining this part of the heavens, there seems to be no other star that could be alluded to, except κ Draconis. About 1326 B.C. this star was within four degrees of the pole, which was sufficiently near to make it appear immoveable to such observers. But from the discordant positions of the stars assigned by Eudoxus, it is inferred that little dependance can be placed on him; and if Eudoxus copied any very ancient sphere, it must have been one of Oriental origin." Hist. of Astron. p. 20.

In the same manner Pythagoras, who we have seen travelled in Egypt and the East, likewise resembles the Hindoos in his metaphysical doctrines. It is remarkable also, that he should be thought to have discovered the celebrated properties of the right-angled triangle, as these have long been known to the Hindoos, and which it is proper to add, they "demonstrate in a very singular way, which partakes more of the nature of algebraic reasoning than of pure geometry." The properties of numbers, always a favourite speculation with the Brahmans, was also entered into by Pythagoras; and as he likewise treated of music, so we find it one of the subjects included in the ancient Vedas. In like manner, the revolution of the earth upon its axis, promulgated by Pythagoras, was also entertained by Aryabhatta, one of the ancient Hindoo astronomers. The Pythagorean doctrines respecting comets being as ancient as the universe; revolving round the sun; and visible only in a certain part of their orbit; is exactly similar, as related by Seneca, to that entertained by the Chaldeans, according to Apollonius Myndius, who professed to have studied under them. (Hist. Astr. p. 14).

Thales is the last of the philosophers necessary to mention, as the earliest (B.C. 600) reported to have travelled in the East; also because he is considered the founder of astronomy among the Greeks. Many of his doctrines, however, like those of some of his successors, resemble those of the Hindoos, as he, like them and Pythagoras, considered the earth to revolve upon its axis. To him also is ascribed "the invention of the zodiac, the discovery of the obliquity of the ecliptic, of the tropical revolution of the sun, and the principal circles of the celestial sphere." But it has already, as appears to me, been justly observed, that "many things seem to prove that the science of Thales was of Eastern origin, and that what have been called his discoveries, were doctrines borrowed from Chaldea or Egypt." This is sufficiently evident from the Grecian zodiac being the same as the Egyptian, Chaldean, and Indian; the last remarkable, as having its twelve signs taken from among the twenty-seven lunar mansions. To his followers is also ascribed the fixing of the obliquity of the ecliptic, like the Hindoos, at 24°; so also the invention of the gnomon, which Herodotus, however, says, was borrowed from the Babylonians. But Thales having, after his travels, been able to predict an eclipse of the sun, (referred by Mr. Bailly to the year 610 B.C.,) appears quite decisive of the subject, as of the fact there can hardly be a doubt. He could not have done so without a long series of observations; and these had been made by the nations among whom he travelled, and who had long been able to foretell eclipses. He is reported, indeed, to have learnt the mode from the Egyptians, and to have taught them how to ascertain the height of the pyramids by the length of their shadows.

In addition to this may be mentioned the mode, according to Apuleius, which Thales adopted for determining the apparent diameter of the sun, as this is conformable to the Hindoo practice of expressing the radius in parts of the circumference (v p. 163); for Thales, according to Apuleius, determined the magnitude of the sun, in parts of its own orbit: "now $\frac{1}{720}$ part (which it was stated to be by another author) of a great circle, is 30′: the real diameter of the sun may be taken at a mean, not far from 32′; so that we see the measure of Thales was a good approximation for those early times." (Hist. of Astr. p. 19.)

Considering therefore the sudden introduction of so much new information, and by those who avowedly travelled in quest of it; also that many circumstances concur in proving, that the Orientalists did possess similar information on the same subjects, we can hardly avoid admitting, that much of it was learnt in the regions where these early philosophers travelled. But with our present knowledge we should find it impossible to apportion their respective shares of discovery to each of the nations from whom it may have been learned, as Egyptians, Chaldeans, Babylonians, Persians, Indians, or Chinese. We only know that the Hindoos do possess much of the above information, in their early cultivated and classical language, and that ancient writers give them credit, as well as the Egyptians and Chaldeans, for having cultivated some of the sciences, and made advances in philosophy.

Conformably to the method adopted with some other nations, it will be proper to conclude this account of the Hindoos with such notice respecting their chronology as may enable us to appreciate the probability of their having been a literary and scientific people, at the early periods required to establish their claims to originality. The quotations by Arabian writers, from Hindoo works, and the mention by name of Hindoos, is sufficient to establish the priority of the latter. In Greek and Latin authors of the period of the commencement of the Christian era, the numerous notices of Indian products, indicate, according to the view we have taken, the existence of a resident and observant people. This, however, was the case at much earlier periods, as we know from the embassy of Megasthenes and Onesicritus to the Court of Chandragupta at Patna, B.C. 315. So, Alexander the Great encountered on the frontiers of India powerful nations and civilized people, whose sages had even then acquired a character for wisdom ; their books were sought for, and, if there be any truth in the tradition, (v. p. 158), sent by Callisthenes to Aristotle. In the time of Theophrastus, or 300 B.C., the knowledge of India was more accurate than even in later times ; while even in Hippocrates, or 150 years earlier, we find notices of many Indian drugs. Ctesias, who was a contemporary, had obtained some knowledge of India by his residence at the Persian Court ; through which channel, or by that of Egypt, and with both we have shown that the Greeks held constant communication, a knowledge of Indian products might have been communicated to the West.

The above period, or that of Ctesias and Hippocrates, is only a century posterior to the times when there seems to have been considerable mental activity, with cultivation of literature, among all the nations of the East. Then Buddhism rose in the plains of India ; Pharaoh Nechao reigned in Egypt, and is thought to have circumnavigated Africa by means of the Phœnicians ; while Zoroaster flourished in Persia, and Confucius in China. But we have no means of ascertaining when Sanscrit literature first became known to the Chinese, though we know that there was considerable intercourse between India and China previous to the Christian era.

Hence, there would appear little difficulty in admitting, even if we were without positive testimony, that the Indians might, like other Oriental nations, even at that time have made some advances in the literature and the science which we find treasured up in their sacred language. This would, moreover, account for the perseverance with which Grecian sages travelled in Eastern regions, even from the early time of Thales, or 600 years before the Christian era.

But from our cursory view of ancient commerce, we have seen that from the earliest times it embraced the products of India, which are mentioned by Herodotus, and were sought for by the Phœnicians, whose most flourishing period was from 1000 to 556 B.C. They were used by the Israelites in large quantities in the time of Solomon, or 1000 years B.C.; but they are mentioned at still earlier periods. We have, moreover, seen that the Egyptians, who existed as a powerful and civilized nation under the Sesostridæ, from B.C. 1600 to 800, and were ruled over by the Hyksos from 1800 to the former period, seem in very early ages to have been acquainted with the products of India. There is also a most remarkable resemblance between them and the Hindoos, unaccountable, if we do not admit that these were contemporaries; and therefore if the latter did not originate, must have borrowed the practices which form the points of resemblance, necessarily at times quite incompatible with their also copying from the comparatively modern Arabs, or even from their chief masters, the more ancient Greeks. The only difficulty, therefore, which I feel, is in disbelieving that the Hindoos were an early civilized people; as in this way only can be explained the numerous facts alluded to in the previous parts of this discourse.

Seeing, therefore, that Buddhism, called a reform of the abuses of Brahmanism, arose in the plains of India, at least in the sixth century before Christ, it proves the long anterior existence of the religion of the Brahmans, as well as of the Vedas, in which its doctrines are explained, and which contain no traces of Buddhism, or of the worship of Rama and Chrishna, as these succeeded that of the Elements. But even the Vedas, or at least the fourth, (which is however acknowledged to be posterior to the others,) contains notices of some of the sciences, and among others of that of medicine. As it is admitted also, that the Hindoos must have paid attention to astronomy as early as 945, 1180, and 1425 B.C. (v. p. 149) it is evident that they must then have been a resident and settled people. So far, therefore, from its being improbable, that the activity of mind which had been displayed in the cultivation of one science, should be similarly exerted in prosecuting others, it is almost a necessary consequence of the investigation of one set of phenomena, that the reflective mind should be similarly directed to that of others. Hence supposing the correctness of the opinion of this early cultivation of astronomy and philosophy, as displayed in the Vedas; we should have much greater difficulty in explaining the anomaly which would present itself in the apparent glimmerings of one science, in the midst of so much mental darkness respecting others. Instead of this, we have a full and continued stream of light, which shows that the ancient Hindoos, with great acuteness and philosophical discernment, turned their attention successfully to almost every department of human knowledge, as Language and Literature, Science, and both the Fine and Useful arts. Our great difficulty consists in assigning to their authors, the dates at which they wrote; from their having themselves neglected the important subject of chronology, or from this having been mystified by their short-sighted followers.

Hence it really appears more probable, that the dates assigned to the principal works by the majority of Orientalists, are nearer the correct ones, than the modernised eras which have been conjectured on such apparently insufficient grounds.. The age of Vikramaditya, which is remarkable for the cultivation and patronage of both literature and science, may therefore be considered as correctly determined in having preceded the Christian era by fifty-seven years. The two great poems, the Ramayana and Mahabharat, having been then revised and rearranged, must necessarily have been composed a few centuries previously. Of these, the former is interesting, as containing a notice of Aghastier, the first translator into Tamul of Sanscrit medical literature. The Vedas have undoubtedly a long anterior date, and are supposed to have been composed near fifteen centuries B.C.; and though the fourth is subsequent to the others, it must also be very ancient; and is interesting to us, as containing the Ayur Veda, or the earliest of the medical writings of the Hindoos. For cultivating the sciences, and the production of the above works, there is sufficient time, if we take Hindoo history after the settlement in India, even on the moderate computations which have been determined by the several authors who have investigated the subject. These, omitting the long list of sovereigns of the fabulous ages of Hindoosthan, yet find that the two solar dynasties must have been settled in Oude and Tirhoot, at least from 1500 to 2000 years before the Christian era; while the lunar race, who reigned in Benares, and afterwards in Behar and Delhi, must be equally ancient. Some authors, however, consider both much, or 1000 years, more ancient than the higher of the above dates; and Sir Wm. Jones concludes, that the second or silver age of the Hindoos was subsequent to the dispersion from Babel; and that we have only a dark interval of about a thousand years, which were employed in the settlement of nations, the foundation of empires, and the cultivation of civil society.

* Having taken a view of the objects of a course of Lectures on Materia Medica and Therapeutics, as well as a cursory survey of their History, I come now to the third division of my subject, that is, the best mode of studying, as well as of teaching them. Though this is a subject I shall afterwards have to detail, you cannot but allow, considering only the multitudinous details to be collected and arranged, that, the task which I have undertaken is one, at least, of considerable labour. Knowing, however, that difficulties were never yet surmounted by those who had not the courage to encounter them, so I have not attempted to conceal from you, or from myself, the extent of the field to be traversed, though called upon to describe its varied riches and multiplied uses, before there has been scarcely time enough to take a survey of its boundaries. I hope, nevertheless, by attention to method, and by determined industry, to be able to bring together sufficient of what is necessary, with enough of what is new, to ensure that your time may not be mis-spent. Hearing me dilate upon the extent and difficulties of the subject, it will perhaps have occurred to you to have heard Materia Medica and Therapeutics stated as the most easily treated department of the Medical curriculum. I know not whether this be from the limited view that is taken of the subjects which they embrace, or from the high qualifications of the present members of the profession; but I feel my own burden much increased by the way in which these subjects are now taught by my friends, Drs. Thomson and Christison, Mr. Pereira, and others.

The multitude of subjects necessarily embraced will be obvious to any one consulting any of the standard works on Materia Medica and Therapeutics, as our Pharmacopœias and Dispensatories, both English and American, with our

* Here the Lecture is resumed as originally delivered.

several authors, only from the time of Cullen; or such works, as those of Cottereau, Guibourt, Fée, Richard, Merat and De Lens, with Bayle, Barbier, Trousseau and Pidoux, Martius, Esenbeck and Ebermeier, Geiger, Göbel and Kunze, Brandt and Ratzeburge.

The difficulties of treating the subject are, however, I conceive, considerably increased by the position at present occupied by Materia Medica and Therapeutics in the prescribed course of Medical Education. Considering that these presuppose some knowledge of Natural History and Chemistry, as well as of Physiology and Pathology, that we may understand the meaning of terms employed in description, as well as the Natural classifications in which the different substances are arranged; besides their mode of action on the living system, as well as their application as medicines in the treatment of disease; one would not expect to find Materia Medica and Therapeutics placed in the first year of the prescribed course of Medical Education; though, perhaps, it is at present unavoidable, from the short time allotted to medical study. The above opinion has been already expressed by others, and therefore I myself venture to bring it forward, particularly as it has the sanction of a name as high as any in English annals, when we consider his triple claim on Literature, on Science, and on Medicine. I mean that of the late Dr. Young, who, in laying down, in his "Medical Literature," what he considered to be the most judicious course of Education, defers attendance on a course of Materia Medica until the third year of study. The only mode, at present practicable, of avoiding the inconveniences of bringing forward at once so many points, in connexion with each particular subject, is to divide the course into two portions; in the first of which, the several substances may be treated of as objects of Natural History; and in reference to their Physical characters and Chemical composition, with only brief notices of their Physiological action. Thus, after noticing the nature, the physical and sensible properties of the substances constituting medicines; the elements of Pharmacy may be treated of, describing first the Mechanical, and afterwards the Chemical operations of that department of our subject, with the different forms in which medicines are administered, as well as the surfaces to which they are applied. That the terms may be intelligible, which, even in this mode of treating the subject, are necessarily employed in describing each article; it will be necessary to follow the above, with a few lectures on the different modes in which medicines act; as well as the classes in which they are arranged, when considering them only with respect to their Therapeutical uses. We shall then be prepared to enter on the substantive part of the course, and may commence with the Inorganic, and proceed to the Organic kingdom of Nature, or from the Mineral to the Vegetable and Animal kingdoms; introducing under each substance the several Pharmaceutical Preparations, of which it forms the principal ingredient, or from which they derive their names.

In the second portion of the course, the Physiological action of Medicines may be more fully entered upon, in conjunction with their Therapeutical uses; when the several substances which had been treated of according to Natural History classifications, will be arranged with reference to their properties as agents for the cure of disease. This part of the course may be fitly preceded by general observations on the important subjects of Climate, Regimen, Diet, and concluded with others on the Theory and Art of Prescribing.

Having alluded to difficulties, it would ill become me, however, to be alive only to these, sensible as I am of the several advantages of my position. Among these, I would particularly mention the easy accessibility to colleagues, willing and able to aid with their advice and assistance; as well as to varied and increasing Libraries and Museums, Collections of Diagrams and Drawings, and also to a Laboratory and Herbarium; to these, I hope, my own Herbarium and Collection of Materia Medica will be no useless addition for the purposes of illustration. But, as first in value, and sufficiently so to be ranked by itself, I would mention the munificent donation of a Museum of Materia Medica, which I understand is to be a counterpart of their own, by the Society of Apothecaries.* Words are inadequate for expressing the value to us of such a gift: but as a Botanist, I cannot but feel pleased that it should have come from a Body, who have for two centuries patronised my favourite study. As Member of an Institution, called into existence by the exigencies of modern times, I hardly know how sufficiently to appreciate the patronage of those, who have so long and so successfully laboured for the improvement of the general members of the profession, on the only sure basis, that of extended and efficient education. I trust we may take this as an omen of King's College being so considered, because it offers to youth of every calling, opportunities of laying deep the foundations of Literature in conjunction with Religion, and on a basement of Mathematical and Physical Science, raising a Professional superstructure, which will be as creditable to themselves as beneficial to the public.

In conclusion, I have to request your attention to a

* This collection has been received since this Lecture was delivered, and is deposited, with a set for the use of Students, in one Museum, with the Collections of Botany, Mineralogy, and Geology. The other Museum alluded to, contains the Collections of Zoology and Comparative Anatomy, in connexion with those of Human and Morbid Anatomy.

remark, though relating only to myself; and this is to remind you, that the difficulties of a first course on any subject are materially increased, if they co-exist, as they do in my own person, with the first time of lecturing at all. That facility of communicating information, usually only the result of experience, will therefore, I fear, be wanting; but labouring to avoid prolixity, I shall endeavour to be full; and I trust I may escape being superficial, when I wish to be brief. The almost necessary failings which, with the best endeavours to avoid, will still exist, require that consideration, which, on a first course, it is usual and becoming to bestow. More than that it would be unbecoming in me to ask, and injustice, both to yourselves and the Institution to which I have the honour to belong, for you to grant.

*** While these last pages have been passing through the press, some observations by my friend, Mr. Prinsep, Secretary of the Asiatic Society, have arrived, "on the very great similarity between the old Sanscrit and the Greek character, more palpable the farther we retire into antiquity, the older the monuments we have to decipher; so that we might almost advance, that the oldest Greek (that written like the Phœnician from right to left) was nothing more than Sanscrit turned topsy turvy."

The connexion of the Greek with the Phœnician and Samaritan alphabets has been admitted as a strong evidence, that "the use of letters travelled progressively from Chaldea to Phœnicia, and thence along the coasts of the Mediterranean;" (Pantographia, p. 107.) The Greek language has besides been now indisputably proved to be but a branch of the Sanscrit stem.

As Mr. Prinsep's arguments are solely those of graphic similitude and ocular evidence, he has printed the letters of the two alphabets in parallel columns. Of the Greek vowels the majority, and in the consonants every one of the letters, "excepting those of after-invention, are represented with considerable exactness," by the several corresponding letters of the oldest Sanscrit alphabet, "although there is hardly a shadow of resemblance between any two in their modern forms." "Whether the priority is to be conceded to the Greeks, the Pelasgians, or the Hindoos, is a question requiring great research, and not less impartiality, to determine." Journal Asiat. Soc. of Bengal, May 1837, p. 391.

ADDENDUM.

It has been mentioned at p. 64, that Professor Dietz had already discovered, though the fact was unknown to the Author, that the later Greek physicians were acquainted with the medical works of the Hindoos, and that Hindoo physicians even held appointments at the court of Harun-al-Rashid. Mr. Cureton has since published a paper on the Indian physicians at Bagdad, to which Professor Wilson has appended remarks, identifying many of the names. He comes to the conclusion, as the Author had done by another series of proofs, "that the astronomy and medicine of the Hindoos were cultivated anteriorly to those of the Greeks, by the Arabs of the eighth century." Vide Journ. Royal Asiat. Soc. No. XI. p. 105, 1840.

The early attention paid by the sovereigns of India to the culture of trees and of useful plants, and the great attention paid by the natives of India to medicine, and the esteem in which it was held, are proved by the following most important inscription, of the date of about 220 B.C., deciphered by my late friend, the deeply lamented Secretary of the Asiatic Society of Calcutta, Mr. James Prinsep. Journal Asiatic Society, vol. v., p. 158. Calcutta, 1838.

"Everywhere within the conquered provinces of ràja PIYADASI, the beloved of the gods, as well as in the parts occupied by the faithful, such as *Chola, Pida, Satiyaputra,* and *Ketalaputra,* even as far as *Tambapannì* (*Ceylon*),—and moreover within the dominions of ANTIOCHUS the Greek, (of which ANTIOCHUS' generals are the rulers)—everywhere the heaven-beloved ràja PIYADASIS' double system of medical aid is established;—both medical aid for men, and medical aid for animals; together with medicaments of all sorts, which are suitable for men, and suitable for animals. And wherever there is no (such provision)—in all such places they are to be prepared, and to be planted: both root-drugs and herbs, wheresoever there is not (a provision of them), in all such places they shall be deposited and planted.

"And in the public highways, wells are to be dug, and trees to be planted, for the accommodation of men and animals."

2.

THE WELLESLEY DESPATCHES.—INDIA.

THE DESPATCHES, MINUTES, AND CORRESPONDENCE OF THE MARQUESS WELLESLEY, K.G.

During his Administration in India.

Revised by His Lordship, and Edited by Mr. MONTGOMERY MARTIN.

Now complete in 5 large vols. 8vo. with Portrait, Maps, Plans, &c.

Price £6. 10s.

"This is a publication of peculiar and extraordinary interest. The whole of the brilliant policy which ended in crushing the great enemy of our Indian Empire among the native powers, in restoring our political influence with the other courts, and in extinguishing that of France in the East, is here laid before our eyes in every part of its progress: we have the whole history of the events given with a degree of authority and particularity of which there is no other example."—*Edinburgh Rev.*

"The despatches may truly be called national records, of which England may justly be proud, and the very best materials for history, if it be not history itself. Not only do those documents throw almost in every page new lights upon imperfectly known subjects, but they give us fresh facts, with all the multiplicity of their remote causes. They tend to do infinite honour to the noble Marquess, whose wise government they so well illustrate."—*Metropolitan Magazine.*

"The despatches of the Marquess Wellesley are a fine course of political science, detailed in the language of an orator. The letters and papers of the Marquess are of the Wellesleyan stamp; they are masterly."—*New Monthly.*

"Our conviction of the great importance of these valuable papers has been confirmed by every volume we have examined. High as we have always esteemed the statesman-like qualities of Lord Wellesley, we never, till reading this collection of his Indian despatches, had so distinct a notion of the consummate ability and admirable sagacity with which he applied the science of politics to the very peculiar exigencies of British India at the period of his administration. We are not surprised at the high testimony borne by the Court of Directors of the Honourable East-India Company to this work, which, we repeat, is not only a rich treasure of historical facts, but also a mine of political wisdom."—*Asiatic Journal.*

"The volume before us completes the celebrated publication to which it belongs—a publication which is destined to continue a standard contribution to English history, in that most wonderful department of the Empire's relations which has Hindostan for its theatre."—*Monthly Review.*

"This most valuable publication will long be consulted not only for the clear historical light it throws upon the important affairs of the East, during an epoch of intense interest, but as a manual for diplomatists and statesmen. It exhibits the Marquess of Wellesley in strong colours, as a man well and wisely chosen to fill the high station, and meet the vast responsibilities of Governor of India; and while our admiration rises as we read every new proof of his acuteness, sagacity, and talent, we breathe a prayer that the welfare of England may never be perilled by the administration of her affairs being entrusted to incompetent hands."—*Literary Gazette.*

"The despatches of Lord Wellesley are elegant compositions, and the collection is not only valuable as affording the best materials for Indian history, but it is an excellent guide and authority for military officers and civilians who may be employed in the East. The volumes are edited with great care, and do credit to Mr. Martin."—*Naval and Military Gazette.*

"This work cannot fail to command attention. The space which the noble Marquess long filled in the political world—the prominent positions he maintained—the great objects he achieved—the wisdom and foresight which he displayed for so many years in the most important and varied characters—all give weight to this publication, in the pages of which will be traced the workings of a master-mind, through a period of the greatest interest to the British nation."—*John Bull.*

"The despatches of the Marquess Wellesley embrace the most important period in the history of British India. His lordship had to encounter difficulties which would have baffled a less able statesman; but the despatches show us the sound judgment with which his lordship directed the combined movements of the British powers."—*Athenæum.*

3.

HISTORY OF THE POLITICAL AND MILITARY TRANSACTIONS IN INDIA,

During the ADMINISTRATION of the MARQUIS of HASTINGS, From 1813 to 1823. Enlarged from the Narrative published in 1820.

By HENRY T. PRINSEP, Esq., of the Bengal Civil Service.

2 vols. 8vo., with Maps and Plates, £1. 12s. cloth boards, lettered.

4.

The EAST-INDIA GAZETTEER;

Containing particular Descriptions of the Empires, Kingdoms, Principalities, Provinces, Cities, &c. of Hindostan, and the adjacent Countries; India beyond the Ganges, &c.

By the late Walter Hamilton. 2 vols. 8vo. £1. 12s. cloth boards, lettered.

"We have seldom seen a work of the class so judiciously compiled."—*British Traveller.*

"This work is not like the generality of Gazetteers—a mere Dictionary of names and terms with laconic explanations—but is replete with full and important details, and the most interesting histories, descriptions, and characteristic sketches."—*London Weekly Review.*

"We are not aware that there is, in fact, any other publication whatever which affords European readers a guide to the general geography of the East."—*Asiatic Journal.*

5.

PAPERS RESPECTING THE

CULTIVATION AND MANUFACTURE OF COTTON-WOOL, RAW SILK, AND INDIGO.

Printed by order of the East-India Company. 8vo. 12s. cloth boards.

6.

FIRST IMPRESSIONS

And STUDIES from NATURE in HINDOSTAN;

Embracing an Outline of the Voyage to Calcutta, and Five Years' Residence in Bengal and the Duáb, from 1831 to 1836.

By Thos. Bacon, Lieut. of the Bengal Horse Artillery.

2 vols. 8vo. with Plates. £1. 10s. cloth boards.

"This is a very pleasant work; one no less meritorious for the beauty of its illustrations than it deserves our praise for the easy elegance of its style."—*Metropolitan Conservative Journal.*

"To those who are fond of descriptions of Oriental magnificence, anecdotes of tiger-hunting and bear shooting, accounts of the marvellous things with which India is filled, and narratives of perilous and humorous adventures, these volumes will be found a rich storehouse of amusement and instruction."—*Times.*

"Lieut. Bacon's work is just what we should expect and desire. These 'Impressions,' in short, will add to the knowledge and solicitude that exist in this country regarding Hindostan."—*Monthly Review.*

"Mr. Bacon describes his Impressions pleasantly and vividly"—*Tait's Magazine.*

"He possesses a quick eye for the points of character and manners, and the power of telling what he sees, observes, thinks, or hears, in a manner humorous and lively."—*Spectator.*

"We have seldom perused volumes more richly deserving of popularity."—*Weekly Dispatch.*

"We are so well pleased with Lieut. Bacon's 'First Impressions,' that we should have no objection to receive from his pen other two volumes, by way of Second Series."—*Observer.*

"It bears the impress of fidelity on the face of it. Eschewing pedantry, and delivering an unvarnished tale, in plain though lively language."—*Asiatic Journal.*

"His work is embellished with a number of views of striking scenery; the whole is light and entertaining."—*Literary Gazette.*

"Valuable for the new facts concerning India. It is written vigorously."—*Atlas.*

"To Indians at home and abroad, these volumes will be most welcome."—*Naval and Military Gazette.*

"A happy combination of correctness and gaiety. They display an intelligent, acute, and observing mind, and are written in a style which can hardly fail to render them extensively popular."—*Eclectic Review.*

"Lieut. Bacon has a keen eye for beauty in nature,—tells his adventures with gaiety and graphic power."—*Monthly Magazine.*

"As clever an artist as he is an entertaining writer. We confidently recommend the Work to all who are desirous of information blended with amusement."—*Exeter Gazette.*

"A large supply of interesting matter, commingled with so much lively narrative, that what is new is delightful, and what has been in any measure anticipated is made to assume the welcome features of perfect novelty.—Beautifully illustrated with a number of lithographic views."—*Taunton Courier.*

"We recommend the work with great sincerity to all classes of readers."—*Western Luminary.*

"The graphic illustrations of this work are creditable to Mr. Bacon's taste and skill as an artist."—*Athenæum.*

7.

THE EASTERN SEAS; OR, VOYAGES and ADVENTURES in the INDIAN ARCHIPELAGO in 1832, 1833, and 1834;

Comprising a Tour of the Island of Java,—
Visits to Borneo, the Malay Peninsula, Siam, &c.;
Also, an Account of the Present State of Singapore, with Observations on the Commercial Resources of the Archipelago.

By GEORGE WINDSOR EARL, M.R.A.S. 1 vol. 8vo. 12*s.* cloth boards.

"Mr. Earl's volume merits, and will obtain, no ordinary share of attention. The facts detailed, and the suggestions offered in its pages, are calculated to arrest the views and awaken the efforts of merchants, legislators, and philanthropists, in such a way as promises to guide to the most beneficial results."—*Monthly Review.*

"The volume contains much that is novel, communicated in an unaffected and agreeable manner."—*Athenæum.*

"This enterprising and intelligent traveller brings before us very interesting accounts of parts in the Eastern Seas very little known. The entire work is extremely well worth the public attention."—*Literary Gazette.*

"The distinguishing character of Mr. Earl's unpretending book is reality and distinctness."—*Spectator.*

"The author is an intelligent traveller, upon whose accuracy the utmost reliance may be placed. His volume contains much novel information regarding the Dutch and the Arab adventurers in the Eastern Archipelago. His opinions of Java are particularly deserving the attention of our merchants and the Government."—*Naval and Military Gazette.*

"The volume must certainly be useful to all who take an interest in the trade, the statistics, or the history of the islands in the Indian Archipelago."—*Atlas.*

"This work supplies a desideratum which has been long felt in the study of geography. The description of the scenery, productions, &c. of the various places visited by the author, are exceedingly interesting, as are also his numerous remarks on the occupations, customs and manners, religion, &c. of the inhabitants."—*Liverpool Standard.*

"Those who take an interest in the narrative of voyagers, and those engaged in Eastern commerce, will read this book without our prompting."—*Shipping Gazette.*

8.

SCENES AND CHARACTERISTICS OF HINDOSTAN,

With Sketches of Anglo-Indian Society.

By EMMA ROBERTS, Author of "Memoirs of the Rival Houses of York and Lancaster," "Oriental Scenes," &c.

Second Edition. 2 vols. post 8vo. 18*s.* cloth boards.

"We believe that these pages contain the most accurate sketches ever taken of the English in India. Miss Roberts came to the task with unusual advantages, and the result is a most charming work, which only requires to be known to be universally popular."—*Literary Gazette.*

"This is the work of a lively and clever lady; shrewd in all social and domestic matters, with an eye for the picturesque, and a taste for whatever is striking and peculiar."—*Athenæum.*

"Miss Roberts has charmed us by her brilliant and close observing work on India: the evidence of truth and reality is impressed on every page, and connected as English society is with India, the publication of these volumes is a national benefit."—*Lady's Magazine.*

"Never, we think, has British Society in Hindostan, been described with more liveliness and fidelity than by Miss Roberts."—*Tait's Magazine.*

"These pages are full of variety and amusement. The sketches of society are lively and piquant, those of scenery vivid and picturesque; moreover, there is the stamp of truth upon them all. The writer has obviously felt, seen, and understood—three qualifications in which the generality of travellers are deficient."—*Court Journal.*

"To the meagre catalogue of works containing authentic information of European society in India, Miss Roberts has made a very valuable and acceptable addition. Her pictures are all drawn with great spirit and accuracy, and remarkable for the truth of their colouring."—*Quarterly Review.*

"The most thorough knowledge of India, that mere description can impart, will be found in these volumes."—*Metropolitan Magazine.*

"Amusing! graphic! good-tempered! effective! spirited! original! and and yet we have not conveyed an idea of half the enjoyment we experienced from the perusal of these entertaining volumes."—*New Monthly Magazine.*

"It would be great injustice not to praise the execution of this work. Both young ladies who are going out, and old gentlemen who are coming home, may profit by the perusal of these pages."—*Gent.'s Magazine.*

"Being filled with acute observations and conveying much solid information, we refer our readers to it with pleasure, convinced that they will thank us for the introduction."—*United Service Journal.*

"These volumes form a very agreeable, and a very true and complete picture of India."—*Spectator.*

"There is fidelity and character impressed in every one of her pictures."—*Monthly Review.*

9.

BOTANY OF THE HIMALAYAN MOUNTAINS.

ILLUSTRATIONS of the Botany and other Branches of the Natural History of the Himalayan Mountains, and of the Flora of Cashmere.

By J. Forbes Royle, Esq., F.L.S. and G.S., M.R.A.S., &c. &c. &c.

Parts I. to IX., Imp. 4to. 20s. each, with Coloured Plates.

(Part X. will complete the work.)

"We highly recommend this publication to our readers, containing as it does not only an ample store of information respecting the natural productions of the Himalayas, but also the best general view of the physical features of those magnificent mountains with which we are acquainted."—*London and Edinburgh Philosophical Magazine and Journal of Science.*

"We rise from an attentive examination of this work, in doubt whether the botanical knowledge it displays and imparts, or the patriotic spirit which pervades it, calls for the higher admiration."—*London Medical Gazette.*

"A more valuable contribution has rarely been made to the science of Natural History than by the splendid work of Mr. J. Forbes Royle. The prints are beautifully coloured. The work, in short, is highly deserving of public patronage."—*Times.*

"The observations respecting the geographical description of the Flora of Northern India are very interesting; and the work will be valuable in supplying a rich mass of facts on the Natural History (using this term in an extended scale), of a part of the world of which our knowledge has hitherto been very vague and partial."—*Loudon's Gardener's Mag.*

"This magnificent work is already known to almost every botanist in this country, and many more wherever science is courted. If there be any who are ignorant of the riches of description and illustration which it contains, we can assure them that a treasure is in reserve which is most covetable."—*Monthly Review.*

"We may now congratulate the public on a great blank in the physical geography of India being satisfactorily filled up by the appearance of this important work."—*Asiatic Journal.*

"No one who would be acquainted either with the ornamental, the cultural, or the medical qualities of the Indian Flora, can dispense with the possession of Dr. Royle's highly valuable labours."—*Journal of Asiatic Society of Bengal.*

"Mr. Royle's work presents a most systematic and complete view of the natural history of those regions, which, though the first that has been given to the world, will probably long remain the best."—*Mechanic's Magazine.*

"This splendid and beautiful work continues to increase in interest, and will, when finished, become a standard work on the subject which it treats."—*Jameson's Edin. Phil. Journal.*

"The work is chiefly addressed to the scientific naturalist, but contains much that is also interesting to the more general student, as well as a vast number of interesting statements regarding a most interesting portion of the globe."—*Journal of the Royal Geographical Society.*

"Such an authentic and almost official book, in express contribution to an extension of our information, must be welcome, must be valued, must be taken into possession."—*Loudon's Magazine of Natural History.*

"This will be found to be one of the most scientific and comprehensive works of the kind that has ever been published."—*Arboretum Britannicum.*

"The text is rich in original details, as well as in elaborate scientific researches; and every thing bearing on the materia medica, whether as acknowledged in the schools, or as existing only in the unwritten dispensatories of the natives of the country, is studiously noticed."—*British and Foreign Medical Review.*

"A most instructive work."—*Lindley's Introduction to Botany.*

"It is not too much to say of this very remarkable work, that it is indispensable to all who would acquire a knowledge of the vegetation, climate, and soil of the north of India."—*Athenæum.*

"Of this region (the Himalayan) an invaluable account is given by Mr. Royle in the above work, to which we are indebted for the principal part of our data regarding the vegetation of India."—*Penny Cyclopædia.*

10.

CONSIDERATIONS ON

THE POLITICAL STATE OF INDIA.

By Alex. Fraser Tytler, Esq. 2 vols. 8vo. 18s. boards.

11.

MISCELLANEOUS ESSAYS.

By the late H. T. Colebrooke. 2 vols. 8vo. with Plates. £1. boards.

*** The volumes now laid before the public comprise a selection from the several Essays originally published by the Author in the Transactions of the learned Asiatic Societies, with the addition of four Prefaces to works originally edited or translated by him.

12.

MEMOIR OF CENTRAL INDIA,

INCLUDING MALWA AND ADJOINING PROVINCES,

With the History and Copious Illustrations of the Past and Present Condition of that Country.

By Maj.-Gen. Sir JOHN MALCOLM, G.C.B., K.L.S., &c.

Third Edition, with a Map, &c. 2 vols. 8vo. £1. 8s. cloth boards lettered.

"Sir John Malcolm is too well known as a soldier, statesman, and author, to require from us any eulogium. We shall only, in reference to the latter capacity, observe, that his 'Memoir on Central India' is in every respect worthy of his former productions."—*Quart. Rev.*

"The work before us is stamped in every part with the thoughts of a statesman, and the high and honourable feeling of a gentleman."—*British Critic.*

"In recommending this work to the notice of the public, we could not employ terms too strong to convey our high opinion of its great interest, value, and importance."—*Asiatic Journal.*

Also, by the same Author,

INSTRUCTIONS to Officers acting under his Orders

In Central India, A.D. 1821. 8vo. 2s. 6d. sewed.

13.

COLONIAL POLICY OF THE BRITISH EMPIRE.

By the Author of the "History of the British Colonies," &c.

Part I.—GOVERNMENT.

In 8vo. Price 3s. (To be completed in Six Parts.)

"Such a work as this cannot but enlighten and engage all who regard the welfare of the British empire, or of mankind, in no ordinary degree."—*Monthly Review.*

"We recommend it to the notice of all who feel interested in colonial affairs."—*Liverpool Standard.*

"The first of what we are quite sure will prove an admirable series of numbers on a subject of very high importance."—*Atlas.*

14.

HISTORY OF THE INDIAN ARCHIPELAGO.

By JOHN CRAUFURD, F.R.S., late British Resident at the Court of Java.

3 vols. 8vo., with Maps and Plates. £2. 12s. 6d. cloth lettered.

15

OBSERVATIONS ON THE

LAW AND CONSTITUTION OF INDIA;

On the Nature of Landed Tenures; and on the System of Revenue and Finance, as established by the Moohummudum Law and Moghul Government; With an Inquiry into the Revenue and Judicial Administration and Regulations of Police at present existing in Bengal.

By Lieut.-Col. GALLOWAY, of the Hon. East-India Company's Service.

Second Edition, with Additions. 8vo. 12s. cloth boards, lettered.

"The additions made to the present edition of Col. Galloway's valuable work materially enhance its value. These additions are chiefly on the judicial administration, on the police, and on the government of India; the latter of which, indeed, is entirely new."—*Asiatic Journal.*

"A man of sound sense, speaking with the experience of thirty years in India, with opportunities for extensive observation on this head, ought to be listened to with particular regard at this crisis of Indian government."—*Literary Gazette.*

16.

PRODROMUS

FLORÆ PENINSULÆ INDIÆ ORIENTALIS;

Containing Characters of the Plants found in the Peninsula of India; Arranged according to the Natural System.

By ROBERT WIGHT, M.D., F.L.S., &c., Surgeon on the Madras Establishment; and G. A. WALKER ARNOTT, A.M., F.L.S., &c.

Vol. I. 8vo. 16s. boards. (To be completed in two vols.)

"A valuable key to the properties of the vegetable productions of the Indian peninsula, and should form a part of the library of outfit of every medical officer proceeding to India."—*London Medical Gazette.*

"It bears evident traces of extreme care and unsparing labour; and is in our opinion one of the most important works that have been published on Indian botany."—*Jameson's Edin. Phil. Journ.*

17.

CONTRIBUTIONS TO THE BOTANY OF INDIA.

By ROBERT WIGHT, M.D., F.L.S., &c.

8vo. 7s. 6d. boards.

18.

ZOOLOGICAL RESEARCHES IN JAVA

AND THE NEIGHBOURING ISLANDS;

With Coloured Plates, representing Native Quadrupeds and Birds.

By THOMAS HORSFIELD, M.D., F.L.S., &c. &c.

One large vol. royal 4to. £8. 8s. boards.

"This is a valuable work. The plates, by Mr. W. Daniell, are in his best manner, and those containing the anatomical details are superior to any hitherto published in this country. The author appears to be actuated by a sincere and zealous spirit of investigation. What he has observed he has minutely described, and those details are useful, and indeed highly valuable to the scientific."—*Philosophical Magazine.*

"The present work of Dr. Horsfield's discovers several species of animals hitherto unknown to zoologists, and which are not in the large collections at Paris or Leyden. It is formed with much care, and will be of great use in the advancement of natural sciences."—*Bulletin général et universel des Annonces et des Nouvelles Scientifiques.*

19.

SELECT

SPECIMENS OF THE THEATRE OF THE HINDUS,

Translated from the Original Sanskrit;

Together with an Account of their Dramatic System, Notices of the different Dramas, &c.

By Professor H. H. WILSON, of the University of Oxford.

Second Edition. 2 vols. 8vo. £1. 1s. boards.

⁂ The Dramas selected are—The Mrichchakati, or the Toy-Cart—Vikrama and Urvasi, or the Hero and the Nymph—Uttara Rama Charitra, or Continuation of the History of Rama—Malati and Madhava, or the Stolen Marriage—Mudra Rakshasa, or the Signet of the Minister—Retnavali, or the Necklace.

"This work, by one of our most accomplished oriental scholars, is delightful from its novelty; but its true praise is, that it unfolds before us the finest part of a national literature, and thereby illustrates a highly interesting national character."—*Blackwood's Magazine.*

"This is a most important addition to our literature, and will surprise those literary men who were, till now, but little acquainted with the learning of the Hindus."—*New Monthly Magazine.*

20.

MILBURN'S ORIENTAL COMMERCE;

Or, the EAST-INDIAN TRADER'S COMPLETE GUIDE,

Abridged, Improved, and brought down to the present Time.

By THOMAS THORNTON, M.R.A.S.

One vol. royal 8vo., with Maps. £1. 16s. cloth boards, lettered.

*** This valuable work, originally compiled by the late Wm. Milburn, Esq., of the Hon. East-India Company's service, contains a Geographical and Nautical Description of the Maritime Parts of India, China, and neighbouring Countries, including the Eastern Islands, and an Account of their Trade, Productions, Coins, Weights, Measures, Port Regulations, Rates, Charges, &c. &c.

21.

GENERAL

EAST-INDIA GUIDE AND VADE-MECUM,

For the Public Functionary, Government Officer, Private Agent, Trader, or Foreign Sojourner in British India;

Being a Digest of the Work of the late Captain WILLIAMSON, with many Improvements and Additions.

By J. B. GILCHRIST, LL.D. 8vo. 18s. cloth boards, lettered.

"We cannot but recommend this work earnestly to the attention of every young man proceeding to India, as containing more practical information necessary for him to have, than he would be able to obtain in years by merely consulting persons who have resided in the East."—*Oriental Herald.*

"The 'Guide' takes up the youthful adventurer (in nine cases out of ten, a boy from school) at the very outset of his career; informs him what is necessary for his equipment; points out what demeanour is to be observed on board ship, what studies and amusements should be followed; advises how he ought to conduct himself on his arrival in India; warns him against the snares that lie in his path; exhorts to frugality and temperance; and in short enforces, in the most persuasive manner, by exhortation and example, practical wisdom, prudence, and virtue."—*Ibid.*

22.

THE EAST-INDIAN CALCULATOR;

Or, TABLES for Assisting Computation of Batta, Interest, Commission, Rent, Wages, &c., in Indian Money.

By THOMAS THORNTON, M.R.A.S. 8vo. £1. 1s. boards.

*** This work contains copious Tables of the Exchanges between London, Calcutta, Madras, and Bombay, and of the relative Value of Coins current in Hindostan; Tables of the Weights of India and China, with their respective proportions, &c.; also an Account of the Monies, Weights, and Measures of India, China, Persia, Arabia, &c., collected from the best Sources and and latest Authorities.

23.

THE ASIATIC JOURNAL,

AND MONTHLY REGISTER FOR BRITISH AND FOREIGN INDIA, CHINA, AND AUSTRALASIA.

Published on the First Day of every Month. Price 3s. 6d.

*** The *Asiatic Journal* has now been established twenty-one years, and is the only publication which has furnished, during that period, a complete and faithful record of Indian occurrences. The efforts it has made to publish the latest intelligence, and the variety of interesting matter on Oriental subjects of which it is the vehicle, have justly obtained for it an extensive circulation, and rendered it peculiarly valuable to all those who take an interest in Indian affairs, or who have connexions in that quarter.

24.

MINUTES OF EVIDENCE AND REPORT,

Taken before the Select Committee of both Houses of Parliament, 1830.

CHINA TRADE. 2 vols. 8vo. Price £2. 2s. boards.

Also,

REPORT of the Select Committee of the House of Commons on the Affairs of the East-India Company. 8vo. 2s. stitched.

PAPERS respecting the East-India Company's Charter; consisting of the Proceedings of the Court of Directors and Correspondence with His Majesty's Ministers. 8vo. 2s. 6d. stitched.

DEBATES at the East-India House on the Renewal of the East-India Company's Charter. 8vo. 5s. stitched.

25.

INDIA; ITS STATE AND PROSPECTS.

By Edward Thornton, Esq. One volume 8vo. Price 10s. boards.

"We want good elementary books on India—works which convey sound practical information without being overlaid with a mass of superfluous matter. Mr. Thornton's 'India' is precisely such a work."—*Times.*

"We venture to declare, that not one in a thousand of the reading public have anything like the fulness of information regarding India which even a hasty perusal of this volume of 350 pages will convey."—*Monthly Review.*

26.

CONSIDERATIONS RESPECTING THE TRADE WITH CHINA.

By Joseph Thompson, late of the East-India House. Post 8vo. 5s. boards.

"This work throws considerable light upon the intricate question of money exchanges between India, China, and England, bearing more especially upon the remittances to and from Canton."—*Times.*

"This is a seasonable publication, and will contribute in no small degree to the information that is so essential to the whole mercantile community of the United Kingdom, and will doubtless tend to promote the interests of British commerce. It abounds with carefully-considered and many important suggestions for the use of our mercantile classes."—*Monthly Review.*

27.

THE POLITICAL, FINANCIAL, AND COMMERCIAL CONDITION OF THE ANGLO-EASTERN EMPIRE IN 1832.

By R. Montgomery Martin. Second Edition. 8vo. 9s. boards.

Also, by the same Author,

British Relations with the Chinese Empire in 1832.

8vo. 2s. 6d. stitched.

28.

MEMOIRS OF THE OPERATIONS OF THE BRITISH ARMY IN INDIA

During the Mahratta War of 1817, 1818, and 1819.

By the late Lieut.-Col. Valentine Blacker, C.B., of the Madras Army.

4to., with Maps and Plans. £2. 2s. cloth boards, lettered.

29.

SACRED AND HISTORICAL BOOKS OF CEYLON

(The MAHAVANSI, the RAJA-RATNACARI, and the RAJA-VALI);

Also, a Collection of Tracts illustrative of the Doctrines and Literature of Buddhism; translated from the Singhalese.

Edited by EDWARD UPHAM, M.R.A.S. and F.S.A., &c.

3 vols. 8vo. £2. 2s. boards.

"This work of Mr. Upham's contains so much precious information regarding the Philosophical and Literary History of Buddhism, that the critic has great difficulty in making a selection of that portion to which he ought to call the attention of his readers. Letting alone the great number of Oriental works which zealous and learned Englishmen have extended over Europe, it is impossible that the present can be too much appreciated."—*Journal des Savans.*

30.

HASSAN ALI ON THE MUSSULMAUNS.

OBSERVATIONS made during a Twelve Years' Residence in a Mussulmaun's Family in India; descriptive of their Manners, Customs, &c. &c. &c.

By MRS. MEER HASSAN ALI. 2 vols. 8vo. £1. 1s. boards.

31.

CUSTOMS OF THE MOOSULMANS OF INDIA.

By JAFFUR SHURREEF (a Native of the Deccan).

Composed under the direction of, and translated by, G. A. HERKLOTTS, M.D. Surgeon on the Madras Establishment.

One vol. 8vo., 16s. cloth boards, lettered.

*** This work comprises a full and exact Account of the various Rites and Ceremonies of the Moosulmans of India, from the moment of Birth to the hour of Death; including their Fasts and Festivals (particularly the Mohurrum); their Vows and Oblations for every Month in the Year; their different Tribes and Sects, Saints, and Devotees; Religious Tenets, Prayers, and Ablutions; the Calculation of Nativities, Necromancy, Exorcism, Casting out Devils, &c. &c.

"Most decidedly one of the most important works on the Mahomedan religion which has ever yet appeared."—(M. Garcin de Tassy) *Journal des Savans.*

"It fills an important chasm. Its details are exceedingly minute, and of the utmost precision. Besides the amusement to be derived from some of its chapters, there are many others which are interesting; its utility, however, as a book for study and reference, constitute its chief value."—*Times.*

"The information under all the heads is of a most interesting character. We most cordially recommend the volume."—*New Monthly Magazine.*

"It possesses a character of authenticity, and its descriptions of Indian manners and customs are distinguished by an exactness and fulness of observation which no European observer could ever hope to attain."—*Literary Gazette.*

"Never were we more disposed to agree in the justice of the poet's maxim, that 'the proper study of mankind is man,' than after the perusal of the present extraordinary volume."—*Monthly Review.*

32.

THE MYTHOLOGY OF THE HINDUS,

With Notices of various Mountain and Island Tribes who inhabit the two Peninsulas of India and the Neighbouring Islands.

Compiled from the best Authorities, with Plates illustrative of the Principal Hindu Deities.

By CHARLES COLEMAN, Esq. 4to. £2. 2s. cloth boards.

33.

TRANSLATION OF SEVERAL PRINCIPAL

BOOKS, PASSAGES, AND TEXTS OF THE VEDS,

And of some Controversial Works on Brahminical Theology.

By RAJAH RAMMOHUN ROY. 8vo. 7s. boards.

"This is one of the most curious collections that has ever appeared in print; it presents the phenomenon (for it is such, since history gives no similar instance) of a learned Brahmin, instructed in European languages and arts, presenting in London a second edition of his theological and controversial writings, originally published at Calcutta, in Sanscrit, Bengalee, and English, for the purpose of proving to his countrymen, the Brahmins of India, that the Vedas, their sacred books, teach God's unity, and that the ancient written laws of Menu and Dhanavalkya, and others, by no means prescribe the necessity of widows burning themselves on the funeral piles of their husbands: we sincerely admire his character and learning, as well as his writings, which are expressive of the highest intelligence, devoted to the progress and happiness of mankind, as the first link which connects the Eastern and the Western world."—*Revue Encyclopédique.*

"A work well worthy of the attention of those who desire to form a correct estimate of pure Hinduism. We may add, as another recommendation to the work, that it may eventually prove a help to the diffusion of Christianity."—*Times.*

34.

A VIEW OF THE

HISTORY, LITERATURE, AND RELIGION OF THE HINDOOS,

By the late Rev. WM. WARD, one of the Baptist Missionaries at Serampore.

3 vols. 8vo. £1. 16s. cloth boards.

Also, by the same Author,

FAREWELL LETTERS to a few Friends in Britain and America,

On returning to Bengal in 1821. 12mo. 6s. boards.

35.

A HISTORY OF MUHAMMEDANISM,

Comprising the Life and Character of the Arabian Prophet, and succinct Accounts of the Empires founded by the Muhammedan Arms, &c. &c.

By the late CHARLES MILLS, Esq. 8vo. 12s. boards.

36.

THE ROUND TOWERS OF IRELAND;

Or, the History of the TUATH-DE-DANAANS, for the first time Unveiled.

By the late HENRY O'BRIEN, Esq., A.B.

Second Edition. 8vo. £1. 1s. cloth boards.

"This gentleman has produced a theory of a very startling kind. He argues that Iran, or Persia, according to the concurrent testimony of sacred and profane history, was the scene of early civilization and refinement. The Irish, he contends, are descended from Persian progenitors; and in the Irish language, accordingly, we may seek an exposition of ancient creeds, of which the most ancient was that which shrouded, under peculiar symbols, the downfall of our first parents—particularly Buddhism and the Linga worship, of which the celebrated 'Round Towers' are demonstrated to be symbols."—*Asiatic Journal.*

"Mr. O'Brien's Essay will afford a great treat, as much as by what he says collaterally, and the evident bearings of his facts and deductions, as by his resolving the great question—what was the origin and the use of these 'Round Towers?'"—*Globe.*

"To Henry O'Brien belongs the honour of deciding the question of their origin, antiquity, and purpose, with a power whose strength appals us."—*Freemason's Quarterly Review.*

"Proofs drawn from every possible branch of human learning."—*Spectator.*

37.

THE EAST-INDIA REGISTER AND DIRECTORY

(PUBLISHED HALF-YEARLY),

Compiled from the Official Returns received at the East-India House,
By F. CLARK, of the Secretary's Office, E. I. House.

One thick vol. 12mo. Price 10*s*. sewed.
Or the Presidencies separate, *viz.*—Bengal, 6*s*.; Madras, 5*s*.; Bombay, 5*s*.

38.

SYNOPSIS OF PRACTICAL PERSPECTIVE,

LINEAL AND AERIAL.

By T. H. FIELDING, Teacher of Painting in Water-Colours to the Senior Classes at the Hon. E. I. Company's Military Seminary, Addiscombe.

Second Edition, enlarged. Royal 8vo. 24*s*. cloth boards.

39.

A TREATISE ON FORTIFICATION,

WITH A MEMOIR ON ARTILLERY.

By HECTOR STRAITH (Captain h. p. unattached), Professor of Fortification and Artillery at the E. I. Company's Military Seminary, Addiscombe.

Second Edition, in one large vol. royal 8vo., with Atlas. £1. 10*s*. cloth bds.

"A very valuable practical treatise on fortification."—*United Service Journal.*

IMPORTED FROM INDIA.

40.

JOURNAL OF THE ASIATIC SOCIETY OF BENGAL,

From January 1832 to December 1836, price 2*s*. 6*d*. each Number.
From January 1837 to the latest date imported, price 3*s*. 6*d*. each Number.
Edited by JAMES PRINSEP, F. R. S., Secretary of the Physical Class, Asiat. Soc.
Published monthly. (Calcutta.)

Also, by the same,

USEFUL TABLES, forming an Appendix to the above.

Part I. Containing Coins, Weights, and Measures of British India. 8vo. 5*s*.
Part II. Containing a Series of Indian Chronological Tables. 8vo. 7*s*. 6*d*.
Part III. Containing a Tabular View of the Generic Characters of Roxburgh's Flora Indica. 8vo. 6*s*.

41.

MADRAS JOURNAL OF LITERATURE AND SCIENCE,

Published under the auspices of the "Madras Literary Society and Auxiliary Royal Asiatic Society."

Edited by the Secretary to the Asiatic Department.

Vols. I. and II. 8vo. 12*s*. 6*d*. each, or half-bound, 14*s*. 6*d*. each. (Madras.)

42.

CHINESE MONTHLY REPOSITORY,

From May 1832 to the latest date imported. Price 2s. each Number.
Printed at Canton.

43.

ASIATIC RESEARCHES;

Or, Transactions of the Society instituted in Bengal for inquiring into the History, the Antiquities, the Arts and Sciences, and Literature of Asia.

Vols. XIX. Part I., and XX. Part I. Royal 4to. £1. 1s. each.
(Calcutta printed.)

Also, former volumes.

44.

INDEX to the first 18 Volumes of the above.

Royal 4to. 15s. sewed. (Calcutta.)

45.

TRANSACTIONS OF THE

MEDICAL AND PHYSICAL SOCIETY OF CALCUTTA,

With Appendices, containing much valuable Matter, &c.

Vol. I. to VII. 8vo. Each vol. 15s. (Calcutta.)

46.

(Under the auspices of the Government of India, and of the Asiatic Society of Bengal),

THE ARABIAN NIGHTS' ENTERTAINMENTS.

(The 1001 Nights complete.)

In the original Arabic. Now, for the first time, published, under the direction of W. H. MACNAGHTEN, Esq., Bengal Civil Service, V. P. A. S.

4 vols. royal 8vo. boards, price £6. (Printing at Calcutta.)

47.

THE PRACTICE OF COURTS-MARTIAL,

AND OTHER MILITARY COURTS;

With Chapters on Inquests; Courts of Requests; Three Trials (Arson, Larceny, and Murder, with full Evidence); Rules of Evidence; and other Useful Matter and Tables.

By Captain WILLIAM HOUGH, Bengal Army.

8vo. 14s. (Calcutta printed.)

48.

OBSERVATIONS ON THE COLONIES OF

NEW SOUTH WALES AND VAN DIEMEN'S LAND.

By JOHN HENDERSON. 8vo. 7s. boards. (Calcutta.)

Works in the Press.

TRAVELS IN WESTERN INDIA.

By the late Lieut.-Colonel JAMES TOD. Royal 4to.

*** This work, which was left by the Author in a complete state for publication, embraces a highly interesting account of a visit to Mount Aboo, and the holy places of the Jains; a description of the ancient city of Anhulwarra (first discovered by the Author), the capital of the Balhara Sovereigns; and descriptions of Somnath and the Jain temples at Girnar. The graphic illustrations represent some exquisite relics of ancient Hindu architecture.

ANGLO-INDIA, Social, Moral, and Political;

Being a Collection of Papers from the Asiatic Journal. 3 vols. post 8vo.

AN ACCOUNT OF CHINA,

Comprehending its Political History, Government, Laws, Literature, Institutions, Manners, and Customs;
Its Geography; Commerce, Internal and External;
The Duties and Regulations in respect to Foreign Trade;
An Accurate Account of the Coins, Weights, and Measures, at Canton;
A History of British Intercourse with China, &c. &c. &c.

2 vols. 8vo., with numerous Plates.

SKETCHES OF THE LATER HISTORY OF BRITISH INDIA.

By the Author of "India; its State and Prospects." 8vo.

*** These Sketches embrace the main features of the History of British India, from the death of the Marquess Cornwallis to the termination of the administration of the Marquis of Hastings—a period distinguished by a series of events of great interest and importance.

ILLUSTRATIONS OF THE HISTORY AND PRACTICES OF THE THUGS OF INDIA;

With some Account of the Progress made by the Government of India in their Suppression. 1 vol. 8vo.

AN ALPHABETICAL LIST OF THE OFFICERS OF THE INDIAN ARMY; AT THE THREE PRESIDENCIES;

From the Year 1760 to the Year 1834 inclusive, with their Date of Appointment as Cadet;
Of their respective Promotions; and of their Retirement, Resignation, or Death;
To the Year 1837, whether in India or in England.

Compiled by Messrs. DODWELL and MILES, East-India Army Agents.

Imperial 8vo. Price: Bengal, £1. 1s.; Madras, 15s.; Bombay, 15s.; or the Three Presidencies, in One Vol., £2. 2s.

LONDON, NOVEMBER 1837.

SELECT LIST OF

Maps, Charts, Atlases, &c.

PUBLISHED BY

WM. H. ALLEN & Co.

I.

A MAP of INDIA, from the latest Surveys of the best Authorities, and corrected to the present time. On Six Sheets of Atlas, £2. 12*s*. 6*d*.; on cloth, in a case, £3. 13*s*. 6*d*.; or on cloth, with rollers, varnished, £4. 4*s*.

II.

SMALLER MAP of INDIA, compiled from the latest Documents, on One large Sheet, 18*s*; or on cloth, in a case, or with rollers, £1. 5*s*.; or with rollers, varnished, £1. 9*s*.

III.

MAP of the WESTERN PROVINCES of HINDOOSTAN, constructed from the most recent Surveys. On Four Sheets of Atlas, £1. 11*s*. 6*d*.; or on cloth, in a case, £2. 5*s*.

IV.

A MAP of CHINA and the ADJACENT COUNTRIES, including Corea, part of Japan, the Islands of Formosa, Philippines, &c. On One large Sheet, coloured, 8*s*.; on cloth, in a case, 11*s*.; on cloth, with roller 12*s*. 6*d*.; or varnished, 14*s*.; or in a frame, varnished, £1. 14*s*. 6*d*.

V.

GENERAL CHART from ENGLAND to CHINA, including the Indian Seas; inscribed to James Horsburgh, F.R.S., &c. &c. On One large Sheet, price 7*s*. 6*d*.; or on cloth, bound, 10*s*. 6*d*.; or on cloth, bound and coloured, 12*s*.

VI.

TWENTY-NINE SHEETS of a NEW ATLAS of INDIA, on a Scale of Four Miles to an Inch. Each Sheet, 8*s*.

*** This Atlas is engraving, by order of the Hon. Court of Directors, by Mr. John Walker, from Trigonometrical Surveys made for the purpose, being intended to form a complete Map of the whole of India on an uniform plan. An Index Map, showing the disposition of the sheets, may be seen at 7, Leadenhall Street.

VII.

INDEX, containing the Names and Geographical Positions of all Places in the MAPS of INDIA. 12mo. 10*s*. boards.